The Complete Medical School Preparation & Admissions Guide

Andrew G. Goliszek, Ph.D.

Third Edition

Healthnet Press
PO Box 24906
Winston-Salem, NC 27114

Goliszek, Andrew
    The complete medical school preparation and
    admissions guide / Andrew G. Goliszek — 3rd ed.
    p. cm.
    Includes bibliographical references.
    ISBN: 0-9616475-6-6
    LCCN: 99-67977

    1. Medical colleges – United States -- Admission.
    2. Medical colleges – United States – Entrance requirements
    3. Premedical education.
I. Title

R838.4G65 2000   610'.711'73

Contents

Introduction

You're deciding or have already decided on a career in medicine. If you're like many other students debating whether or not medicine is for them, you're probably a good student, you enjoy science, and you have a strong desire to do something worthwhile with your life. Since many students choose medicine as a career, you can improve your chances markedly if you begin a plan that will get you ready now for that final decision. By starting your preparations as soon as possible, you can avoid the problems many others face when applying to medical school.

Each year, more than 250,000 college freshman register as pre-medical majors, and by their senior year only 40,000 of them are qualified enough to apply for a limited number of places in U.S. medical schools. Sadly, what many of these students don't realize is that grades are not enough and sometimes not as important as other factors. The real key to successful admission is knowing the specific qualities medical schools are looking for and beginning a strategy than can guarantee that admission.

A Self Analysis

Before doing anything else, you need to do some serious soul-searching. Be honest with yourself when answering the following list of questions and try not to be too hasty in your evaluation. The self-analysis you make is important when considering a career in medicine. Don't take it lightly.

Why do you want to be a doctor?

Are you thinking about medical school because it's expected of you?

What is the most attractive aspect of medicine to you?

Are you going into medicine mainly for financial reasons?

Do you have a sense of compassion for people?

Are you honest with yourself, as well as with others?

Are you willing to work long hours in school and continue to work long hours as a physician?

Are you willing to be around sick and dying people?

Are you ready to make personal sacrifices in order to help others?

Are you an understanding person?

Do you have a sincere desire to put up with intolerable conditions at times for the benefit of others?

Are you basically calm and have a reassuring manner?

Are you a good communicator?

Do you get along with all kinds of people?

What qualities do you possess which would enhance a doctor-patient relationship?

As you can see, many of these questions deal with personal qualities a physician must have in his or her dealings with patients and colleagues. If you lack the necessary attributes of compassion, sincerity, understanding and motivation, then medicine is not for you. There are students who attend medical school simply because it will provide them with a lucrative career, but these individuals will probably never attain the genuine satisfaction that comes with knowing that they will be doctors for one reason - to help the sick. The rewards of personal satisfaction and intellectual growth make the difficult years worthwhile.

If you've answered the questions honestly and feel you have the personal qualities that would make you a good candidate, you need to begin preparing yourself both intellectually and socially. In the chapters ahead, I'll discuss ways in which you will increase your chances for success by enhancing both your academic and non-academic credentials.

How To Begin

All too often, students get incomplete advice from counselors who aren't totally familiar with medical school admissions requirements. This is especially true at colleges that don't have premedical programs and, therefore, don't have someone who is intimately aware of premedical academic and non-academic requirements. Sometimes a student is not sure about medical school and doesn't know what information is available. The ideal situation is to pay a visit to a premedical school advisor at your school or at the nearest school that has one. The premedical advisor should be in constant contact with medical schools in the area and their faculty and can give you valuable information about different medical schools and the literature currently available. Talking to an advisor and spending some time reading these publications will start you thinking about the role you need to take in developing your own future.

The key is to begin now. I've talked to many college seniors who regret not having started a plan of action sooner. If there's anything I can't emphasize enough, it's the importance of not waiting until it's too late. The sooner you get started, the better off you'll be. And don't assume that being a good student is enough. Medical schools don't want excellent students who have nothing to show but the fact that they've spent four years studying. Your plan of action needs to include other areas of accomplishment besides academics in order for you to develop into the well-rounded individual medical schools are looking for. The following chapters include much information about what to do and not to do in order to be a successful medical school candidate. I hope they truly enhance your chances for admission and make this a career choice that's right for you.

1

Medical School Education

Variety in Medical School Programs

In general, the time needed to complete the requirements for an M.D. degree is four years. The curricula at each school, though similar, varies in terms of electives, the number and types of required courses, and the time sequence in which students would take those courses. Therefore, what seems attractive to one individual may not be for another. Prospective students need to read each school's catalogue for the most recent changes and additions, and to see how different schools train their doctors in their own ways.

Regardless of the time allotted to coursework and the differences in academic systems, the nature of the curricula is basically the same. During the first two years, there's a focus on the basic sciences. Courses include: Anatomy, Biochemistry, Genetics, Physiology, Pharmacology, Histology, Embryology and Behavioral Science. Again, different medical schools vary in both the order of introducing these topics and the manner in which they're presented to students. Some schools prefer to integrate courses and to interrelate them with the organ systems. Other schools take a more independent approach and teach the courses separately. Whatever the approach, the aim of the curriculum is to prepare the medical student for the final two years of clinical medicine, which emphasize the application of science to the solution of clinical problems.

Teaching philosophies also differ between schools. Here's a statement made to me by a professor of physiology and pharmacology at the medical school with which I'd been affiliated:

"I think of medical school more like a trade school than a university. Students come here to learn a specific trade and must know certain facts in order to qualify to perform that trade. Our purpose is not so much to dwell on theoretical aspects of medicine but rather to give students the tools needed to become physicians. In order to be a physician, you need to acquire an incredible amount of information and facts, and we simply do not have the time to get into much theory during classroom time."

To give you an idea of how much information is given to students during medical school, some students I've talked to form study groups in which one student attends lectures and takes notes, another does the outside readings, and still another organizes study notes and does other academic requirements. These students felt that they would not have had the time to do everything on their own without spending every waking hour studying or reading. Most students, though, learn early on to form good study habits and to cooperate with classmates in order to get through the rigors of medical school with good grades.

Medical school can be a very difficult time for students who lack the desire and motivation to work hard or don't have the necessary attributes to cope with a medical school curriculum. According to studies, an individual must have five qualities in order to ensure success in medical school. These are:

1. Strong motivation
2. Ability to pursue problems in great depth
3. A capacity for sustained scholarship

4. A capacity to think logically and reason clearly

5. A persistent sense of pressure to wonder and seek answers to problems

Having these qualities doesn't necessarily mean that an individual will get through medical school with flying colors. Not having them, however, can mean a great deal of trouble in keeping up with classmates you'll be competing against for spots in residency programs.

Clinical Clerkships

Usually, the last two years of a medical curriculum consist of many clinical clerkships in which students participate in patient care settings. Every medical school requires clerkships in Internal Medicine, Obstetrics-Gynecology, Pediatrics, Psychiatry and Surgery. Some other schools also require clerkships in Family Medicine and surgical specialties. During the clerkships, which last anywhere from four to fifteen weeks each, students are under close faculty supervision and become involved in the process of diagnosis and treatment of actual medical problems. This is also the time when students begin to recognize particular interests and may decide on the specialty they would like to pursue during their residence programs.

The final two years of the curriculum also allow time for electives, which provide additional experience in areas of interest. Electives vary from school to school, and in many schools may comprise the entire fourth year. Grades at most medical schools are awarded as pass/fail, but some schools still retain the letter grade system or the number system, with 1 being the lowest and 4 the highest.

Examples of Medical School Curricula

A catalogue from any medical school will give you an idea of what each school year is like and the kinds of courses and clerkships required. The following four examples are actual curricula from four different medical schools. They illustrate the similarities and differences in a four-year medical education.

School A

1st Year	Biochemistry, Physiology, Gross Anatomy, Micro Anatomy, NeuroAnatomy, Genetics, Pathology, Bacteriology, Pharmacology, Immunology, Clinical Diagnosis, Psychology
2nd Year	Medicine, Surgery, Pediatrics, Psychiatry, Obstetrics-Gynecology, Family Medicine
3rd/4th Year	Electives and Clerkships

School B

1st Year	Biochemistry, Gross Anatomy, Micro Anatomy, Physiology, Pharmacology, Psychology, Pathology, Immunology, Interdisciplinary studies of the Nervous, Respiratory, Cardiovascular, Renal, and Endocrine systems
2nd/3rd Year	Systemic Pathology, Laboratory Diagnosis, Seminars & Conferences, Physical Diagnosis, Clinical Pharmacology, Clerkship Rotations
4th Year	Electives and Rotations

School C

1st Year	Biochemistry, Physiology, Histology, Human Genetics, Biostatistics, Humanities, Radiobiology, Neurobiology, Gross Anatomy, Anatomic Radiation, Molecular Genetics, Cell Pathology, Community Medicine, Behavioral Science, Problem Solving Projects
2nd Year	Microbiology, Pharmacology, Pathology, Health Ecology, Humanities, Psychiatry, Physical Diagnosis, Community Medicine, Clinical Medicine, Problem Solving Projects
3rd/4th Year	Medicine, Surgery, Obstetrics-Gynecology, Psychiatry, Neurology, Selected Clerkships

National Board Examinations

The Federation of State Medical Boards (FSMB) and the National Board of Medical Examiners (NBME) administer a three-step examination, the USMLE, for medical licensure in the United States. Nearly all candidates sit for Parts I and II prior to completion of medical school, and many medical schools use scores in their student evaluation system. Part III is taken following the granting of the MD or DO degree and passing Parts I and II.

According to the American Association of Medical Colleges Curriculum Directory, approximately 75 percent of the 127 accredited medical schools in the United States require their students to take Part I during the academic year. Part II is required of about 70 percent of the schools. Typically, all three parts are completed within a seven-year period which begins when an individual passes his or her first step. The 3 steps of the United States Medical Licensing Examination (USMLE) are:

1. Assessing an applicant's knowledge and understanding of basic biological science, with an emphasis on principles and mechanisms of health, disease, and modes of therapy.

2. Assessing whether an applicant can apply medical knowledge and clinical science considered essential for patient care under supervision, including emphasis on health promotion and disease prevention.

3. Assessing whether an applicant can apply medical knowledge and biomedical and clinical science considered essential for the "unsupervised" practice of medicine, with emphasis on patient management in ambulatory settings.

Candidate pass rates on Parts I and II have consistently been higher than non candidate rates. Annual pass rates in previous years have ranged from 82 to 86 percent for Part I and 97 percent for Part II. For more information on the NBME or the USMLE, write to:

National Board of Medical Examiners	USMLE
3750 Market Street	3750 Market Street
Philadelphia, PA 19104	Philadelphia, PA 19104
Tel: (215) 590-9500	Tel: (215) 590-9600
Fax: (215) 590-9555	Fax: (215) 590-9470

Internships and Residence

An intern is a medical school graduate spending his or her first year out of medical school in residence at a teaching hospital. During internships, graduate medical students continue to develop their skills under the close supervision of a doctor or a team of doctors and are responsible for the actual diagnosis and treatment of patients under their care.

Depending on their interests and plans for a specialty, interns usually spend their first year in a broad and flexible program or enter directly into a specific program. A graduate student choosing to enter general practice rather than specializing would typically spend a year as an intern before starting a private practice or working in a clinic or HMO with a team of doctors.

In 1965, the American Medical Association recommended that the internship be abandoned and that the graduate medical training period be combined instead with the residency. The residency period is one of sustained specialty training. In 1975, all existing internships were incorporated into a combined program designed to meet the requirements of board certification. Students may still choose "flexible" internships, however, which are designed to provide a wide range of clinical experiences during the year following graduation.

Today, most residents don't normally work the long and intolerable hours once considered a necessary part of the residence years, but they still manage to put in many more hours than the average person does. The hospital work involves shift rotations, which include being on call for periods of time in various departments such as the emergency unit, obstetrics, pediatrics, surgery, and the intensive care unit. In return for their services, residents get a salary, benefits and clothing allowing.

A medical school graduate will usually serve his or her residency immediately following graduation, but this isn't a hard and fast rule. Some doctors spend a few years practicing medicine before deciding to serve a residency and becoming certified in a specialty or subspecialty.

Fields of Specialty and Subspecialty

The vast majority of medical school graduates choose a field of specialty prior to completing their M.D. degrees. A few go on to Ph.D. programs if they wish to develop careers as medical scientists and may later try to enter a residency program.

Here is a list of specialties and subspecialties medical school graduates may choose after completion of a four year M.D. degree. Following the description of the specialty is the average number of years required to serve that residency in order to become certified. There may be some differences in residency length from state to state, but in general the time required is the same.

Allergy & Immunology

Diagnosis and treatment of various allergies and diseases associated with the immune system.
Subspecialty: Clinical & Laboratory Immunology
Residence length: 2 years

Anesthesiology

Administration of anesthesia prior to and during surgery.
Subspecialties: Critical Care Medicine, Pain Management
Residence length: 4 years

Colon & Rectal Surgery / Proctology

Diagnosis, treatment and surgical management of diseases of the colon and rectum.
Residence length: 1-2 years

Dermatology

Diagnosis and treatment of skin disorders and diseases.

Subspecialties: Clinical & Laboratory Dermatology Immunology, Dermatopathology

Residence length: 4 years

Emergency Medicine

Treatment of emergency cases such as accidents, traumas and immediate life-threatening situations.

Subspecialties: Medical Toxicology, Pediatric Emergency Medicine, Sports Medicine

Residence length: 2-3 years

Family Practice

Diagnosis and treatment of diseases and illnesses of all family members and the general health care of adults and children within the family unit.

Subspecialties: Geriatric Medicine, Sports Medicine

Residence length: 3 years

Internal Medicine

Diagnosis and treatment of adult internal disorders.

Subspecialties: Adolescent Medicine, Cardiovascular Disease, Clinical Cardiac Electrophysiology, Clinical & Laboratory Immunology, Critical Care Medicine, Endocrinology Diabetes and Metabolism, Gastroenterology, Geriatric Medicine, Hematology, Infectious Disease, Medical Oncology, Nephrology Pulmonary Disease, Rheumatology, Sports Medicine

Residence length: 3 years

Medical Genetics

Diagnosis and treatment of genetic-based illnesses and disorders.

Subspecialties: Clinical Biochemical Genetics, Clinical Cytogenetics, Clinical Genetics, Clinical Molecular Genetics

Residence length: 2-3 years

Neurological Surgery

Diagnosis, treatment and surgical management of the brain, spinal chord and nervous system.

Residence length: 5 years

Nuclear Medicine

Use of radioactive materials for diagnostic treatment. Administering radionuclides intravenously to scan brain, skeleton, liver, bone marrow, etc. for tumors, diseases and other abnormalities.

Residence length: 4 years

Obstetrics-Gynecology

Care and treatment of pregnancy and childbirth or care and treatment of female disorders.

Subspecialties: Critical Care Medicine, Gynecologic Oncology, Maternal & Fetal Medicine, Reproductive Endocrinology

Residence length: 4 years

Ophthalmology

Care and treatment of eye disorders.

Residence length: 3 years

Orthopedic Surgery

Diagnosis, treatment and surgical management of bone, joint, muscle, cartilage and ligament.

Subspecialty: Hand Surgery

Residence length: 5 years

Otolaryngology

Diagnosis, treatment and usually surgical management of disorders of all head cavities.

Subspecialty: Otology/Neurotology, Pediatric Otolaryngology

Residence length: 5 years

Pathology

Study and identification of causes of diseases.

Subspecialties: Blood Banking/Transfusion Medicine, Chemical Pathology, Cytopathology

Dermatopathology, Forensic Pathology, Hematology, Immunopathology, Medical Microbiology

Neuropathology, Pediatric Pathology

Residence length: 3-4 years

Pediatrics

Care and treatment of all aspects of childhood disorders and diseases.

Subspecialties: Adolescent Medicine, Clinical & Laboratory Immunology, Medical Toxicology, Neonatal-Perinatal Medicine, Pediatric Cardiology, Pediatric Critical, Care Medicine, Pediatric   Emergency Medicine, Pediatric Endocrinology, Pediatric Gastroenterology, Pediatric Hematology, Oncology, Pediatric Infectious Disease, Pediatric Nephrology, Pediatric Pulmonology, Pediatric Rheumatology, Sports Medicine

Residence length: 3 years

Physical Medicine & Rehabilitation

Care, treatment and restoration of diseased, injured and defective limbs and other body parts.

Subspecialty: Spinal Cord Injury Medicine

Residence length: 4 years

Plastic Surgery

Surgical management that involves appearance of any body part.

Subspecialty: Hand Surgery

Residence length: 5 years

Preventive Medicine

Specializing in the prevention of diseases within the community, the environment, and industry.

Subspecialties: Aerospace Medicine, Medical Toxicology, Occupational Medicine, Public Health & General Preventive Medicine, Undersea Medicine

Residence length: 3 years

Psychiatry & Neurology

Care and treatment of behavioral and emotional disorders and disorders of the nervous system.

Subspecialties: Addiction Psychiatry, Child & Adolescent Psychiatry, Clinical Neurophysiology, Forensic Psychiatry, Geriatric Psychology, Neurology, Neurology with Special Qualifications in Child Neurology

Residence length: 4 years

Radiology

Use of X-rays to diagnose physical disorders for the purpose of medical treatment.

Subspecialties: Diagnostic Radiology, Radiation Oncology, Radiological Physics, Neuroradiology, Nuclear Radiology, Pediatric Radiology, Vascular & Interventional Radiology

Residence length: 4 years

Surgery

General field of surgical management on any part of the body.

Subspecialties: General Vascular Surgery, Pediatric Surgery, Hand Surgery

Residence length: 5 years

Thoracic Surgery

Surgery involving organs of the chest.

Residence length: 2 years

Urology

Diagnosis and treatment of disorders of the male urogenital and the female urinary tract.

Residence length: 3-4 years

In some cases, medical students choose specialties early on in their education. But in most cases, choosing a specialty turns out to be a difficult and confusing decision. In fact, as many as 75 percent of all medical students change their specialty choice during medical school. The reasons for indecisiveness? Lack of information, equal appeal of several specialties, not really knowing one's interests, and not knowing one's abilities.

In order to encourage medical students to make more intelligent and concrete choices, one study suggested that students follow certain progressive decision-making rules during each year of medical school. First year students need to begin thinking about the decision-making process and prepare themselves for choices. Second year students should learn as much as they can about specialties and think about their own particular interests and abilities. Third year students need to link their interests and abilities to certain fields of medicine and then explore those areas in great depth. Fourth year students must choose among the few specialties they find equally appealing and try to fit one to their own unique talents as individuals. The more a student applies this kind of approach, the easier it should be to finally decide on the particular specialty most closely suited to his or her interests.

For information regarding the time requirements for each residency and details about certification, write directly to:

American Board of Medical Specialties
1007 Church Street
Suite 404
Evanston, Illinois 60201-5913
Tel: (847) 491-9091

2

The High School Years

Are the high school years too early to begin planning for a future in medicine? According to most admissions experts, good high school preparation is essential in laying the groundwork for successful admissions to choice colleges and ultimately to medical school. One of the main reasons for this is that medical school admissions criteria and policies have been continually changing, and medical school applicants of the '90s and beyond will have a much different profile than did applicants a decade ago. A major change foreseen in future admissions decisions will an emphasis on overall preparation in school as well as life experiences. High school, therefore, can be an important foundation from which to build a strong background and begin to accumulate the credentials necessary for admission.

Because of increasingly intense competition, the road to successful medical school admission for many students has to begin during high school. By developing and building certain attributes, characteristics and credentials, even before applying to college, a high school student will not only be better prepared for premedical education, he or she will enter college with a definite advantage over the thousands of other students intent on getting into one of only 124 U.S. medical schools. As more good students learn how to play the admissions game, the importance of high school premedical preparation becomes even more important. Good students who begin early will have an edge and become top candidates.

From my own experiences in dealing with college freshman, I found it extremely important that students get a good start during the first year. I've seen so many freshman start slowly, fall behind, then try to catch up when it's too late. These were basically good students who never really developed the study habits needed to make it through a rigorous college program with the kinds of grades needed for medical school admission. While a biology lab instructor at Utah State University, I became fairly good at predicting within the first few weeks of class which students would do well just by talking to them about how they prepare for exams and how they studied material I had given them. Invariably, the students who did well were the ones who were good high school students and who brought their study skills to college with them. Naturally, by their senior year, they were the ones being admitted to medical schools.

Students with poor study skills sometimes manage to squeeze through and get admitted to medical school anyway. Unfortunately, they pay the price almost immediately. A friend of mine, who at the time was the curriculum director for physiology at a local medical school, told me that the number one problem he sees during the first year is poor or inadequate study and learning skills. These students had never developed the skills to begin with and had been able to get through college with good grades without having to put much effort into studying. This doesn't work in medical school. By learning to study properly and consistently, students will bring good habits with them and be successfully from the start.

Precollege Coursework

In a later chapter, I'll discuss recommended and required college courses for a premedical curriculum. As a high school student, however, you need to prepare yourself now to do well in those courses later on. Remember, it's important to start your freshman year off right in order to stay on track and keep your grades up. By taking certain courses in high school, you'll be much better prepared for a total premedical education. And according to most admissions committee members, a premedical education isn't only science courses, but non-science courses that medical schools believe are important for the development of a well-rounded individual. An added advantage to beginning your course preparation in high school is that you'll do much better on the SAT and enhance your chances of getting accepted into a college with a good record of successful medical school admissions.

The following are my precollege course recommendations. Since most college premedical curriculums are basically the same, these courses should help you whether you decide to go on to Harvard or Yale or stay home and attend your local state college. These courses will also help prepare you for other health-related curriculums such as pre-dentistry, pre-veterinary, pre-nursing, etc. and make your freshman year in college a whole lot easier.

Recommended Science Courses

Biology - College freshman learn quickly that introductory college biology requires quite a bit of memorization. You'll be subjected to new and often complex terms, ideas and concepts, and I've seen many new students get frustrated at the thought of having to learn so many scientific names and terms. This gets even worse for students taking more advanced biology courses. Students who have taken biology in high school are far more comfortable in college level classes and almost always find them easier and more interesting than do students who've never had high school biology.

Physics - Physics is a required course for any premedical curriculum and usually gives first year students a lot of trouble because they try to take it before they're ready. Like biology, physics is going to include a new set of ideas and terms that you'll be unfamiliar with unless you've introduced yourself to them in high school. A high school physics course, naturally, will be simpler than a college course, but it'll familiarize you with abstract ideas, get you accustomed to basic physics math, and get you thinking in a way that will give you more insight as you learn about more advanced physics concepts. I found that many premedical students either take physics right away because they want to get it over with or put it off because they're afraid of it. Taking a high school physics course will help you overcome that fear and give you an advantage when you get to college.

Chemistry - This subject is the one I feel is most important to prepare for while in high school. Medical schools require one year each of college level biology and physics but two years of chemistry (one year of inorganic and one year of organic). College level chemistry is where most of the premedical students get weeded out, and organic chemistry is probably the most difficult of all the premedical courses for most students. I've heard premedical advisors say that "if you can't get through organic with a B, you won't get into medical school." The reason for that is simple. Many advanced life science classes require a good understanding of organic chemistry. Almost all the students I've known who did well in chemistry have had chemistry in high school. It's easy to get left behind. Begin your college chemistry experience the right way by getting a good foundation during high school.

Advanced Mathematics - Math courses such as algebra and calculus will be very helpful to you regardless of whether you choose to major in biology or business administration. Most medical schools now require at least one college course in college calculus and many require two. By taking advanced math classes, you'll also be much better prepared for physics and chemistry, which require knowledge of at least algebra. Finally, math classes force you to think, and anything that forces you to think in a clear and logical manner will help you in other classes.

Recommended Non-Science Courses

Writing - Almost every college instructor is going to give exams that require some form of essay writing. I've seen good students get poor grades simply because they had poor writing skills, which made exams much harder than they really were. The Medical College Admissions Test has an essay section which determines an applicant's ability to communicate clearly and effectively. Writing skills are recognized by medical schools as important factors in a student's overall academic ability and are adding writing courses to their list of requirements. As a college teacher for many years, I can tell you that you'll definitely be judged by the way you communicate. Those students who write well will almost certainly make a better impression on their teachers and make taking exams much easier. I can also tell you that students who write well will gain their teacher's respect and get the benefit of the doubt on exam questions.

Humanities - The trend in medical school admissions policies and decisions is to recruit well-rounded students with a broad educational base. The time when medical schools accepted science majors almost exclusively is long gone, and according to recent medical journals, humanities subjects need to be put back into premedical education in order to improve the human quality of tomorrow's doctors. Subjects like literature, art, music, etc. are now looked at by medical schools as important factors in helping to improve a student's ability to interact with society and other individuals.

As far as I can see, the trend toward taking more liberal arts and humanities courses will continue and probably increase as medical schools realize that non-science majors do just as well in medical school as science majors do. By taking non-science courses, you'll not only be looked at as more cultured and well-rounded, you'll avoid the dreaded "pre-med syndrome" discusses in the chapter on premedical education. So, without sacrificing basic science courses like biology, chemistry and physics, prepare yourself to be a well-rounded student. You'll not only become a more knowledgeable and interesting person, you'll be doing exactly what medical schools are now expecting you to do if you're really serious about a medical career.

Languages - Most high schools offer foreign languages such as Spanish, French and German. Taking at least two years of a foreign language looks good on your record because colleges feel this makes you a better and more rounded individual. Even though you may never use the language you learn, use this as an opportunity to build your high school credentials and add another feather in your academic cap.

In summary, let's review how you can utilize your high school years to get academically ready for a premedical college curriculum:

1. Improve study and learning skills. Premedical science courses are difficult, and it's essential that you begin college with good study habits and learning skills. Unless you do, you'll be left behind.

2. Improve reading skills. Being able to read with speed and comprehension will make it easier to get through tough courses and enable you to spend more time learning the material.

3. Take science courses that will prepare you for college. Courses I found to be most helpful are biology, chemistry, and advanced math. Students who take these courses in high school seem to be able to grasp the college-level material much better.

4. Take non-science courses such as literature, music and art. Don't think that science is all you'll need to become a top prospect. More colleges and medical schools are reevaluating the importance of humanities and liberal arts in the development of the "total physician."

Choosing the Right College

After talking to many medical school faculty members and medical school admissions officers, I've confirmed one of the most important factors in the selection process - that the undergraduate school you attend has a tremendous impact on your chances for successful medical school admissions. As a high school student wanting to get into medical school, your first goal should be to get admitted to the best college or university you possibly can.

Admissions committees are sometimes notorious for rejecting applicants who've attended small, non-selective colleges in favor of applicants who've graduated from distinguished schools having records of success in placing medical school applicants. One of the main reasons for this is that good colleges with excellent premedical programs tend to weed out students who probably wouldn't make it in medical school. Many small colleges may not even have premedical school advisors, much less entire committees guiding students throughout their first few years in college. Therefore, your first goal needs to be admission into a good college with a good record of success in placing students.

Because the college you attend is a big factor in your chances for acceptance to medical school, you should find out as much as you can about your college choices. Write or call the admissions office or the department that handles the premedical curriculum (usually biology) and find out (insist on) the answers to these questions:

1. What percentage of students who have applied to medical schools from your college have gained admission? Find out the actual number of applicants and the number of successful entrants.

2. What were the academic characteristics (GPA and MCAT scores) of students who've been accepted or rejected by medical schools from your college?

3. What kind of premedical program and premedical curriculum does your college offer?

The reasons for insisting on this information are simple. First, you need to know a school's track record because that's an indication of how medical schools view the undergraduate institution. Naturally, schools with good premedical programs and proven records of placing students who do well in medical school will always have an advantage. Second, the academic credentials of students who do or do not get admitted can give you an idea of a school's reputation. If students with average GPAs are successful in gaining admission to medical school, it's a sure bet that the premedical program is difficult and the level of competitiveness is higher than at other schools. On the other hand, if many students having high GPAs are rejected, the school may not have the reputation of being competitive or selective. Third, a college having an established premedical advisory program can offer you more in terms of preparation and development than one lacking such a program.

Don't be afraid to pursue answers to your questions. Go to or call the admissions office, the premedical advisor, the counseling office, or whoever you need to go for answers. If the school insists that there are no records or information of this kind, or if it refuses to make them available, you should think twice about applying there. Either the school has a bad record of medical school admissions or the premedical program is not well enough run to have that sort of data readily available. A good school with a good record will proudly offer you all the information you need.

Questions About Choosing a College

Here are some of the most frequently asked questions students have when deciding on which college to attend:

Q. Is it better to attend a highly competitive college even though your grades may be lower at graduation?

A. Definitely, yes. Again, medical schools are familiar with college reputations and would rather have a student with a 3.2 GPA from a highly competitive college than a student with a 3.8 GPA from a least competitive school. Your goal should be to get admitted to the most competitive program you can even though your grades might not turn out as good.

Q. Are there any colleges that give students an edge when applying to medical school?

A. Studies have shown that students with the best chances for admission are from "highly selective" private and public institutions. Students from the least competitive schools faired the worst. In fact, the great majority of new entrants come from less than 400 colleges nationwide. So, if your two options are enjoying an easy four years or some very intense ones, definitely choose the latter if you're at all serious about improving your chances for medical school.

Q. Should a student apply to college as a premedical major?

A. Definitely, no. Under no circumstance should you indicate that you're planning to enroll as a premedical student. I've been around college admissions officers and faculty members long enough to know that the term "premed" is an invitation for rejection. The reason: it's not that colleges don't want or need good premed students, it's just that they would rather have good all-around students who may eventually apply to medical school regardless of their major. And since many students never end up in medical school, colleges are on the look-out for students who have alternate career choices. So, never indicate that you plan on being a premed. Once you're accepted, you can major in anything you like anyway.

Q. What's the most important factor that select colleges look for when considering applicants?

A. According to a USA Today survey of nearly 500 college admissions directors, high school grades and the courses in which they were earned are the most important determining criteria. The fact is, A's in tough courses carry more weight than even SAT scores, and the trend now is to look closely at a combination of high grades and the quality of the high school program in order to predict academic success.

Q. Does a student need more than good grades and SAT scores to get admitted into a select college?

A. Yes. Grades and SAT scores alone are not enough. Since the better schools receive thousands of applications from outstanding students, extracurricular activities and distinguishing characteristics definitely help make the selection process more competitive. Not only must you have good grades and SATs, you need to participate in school and community activities, compete in sports and other events, become a member of clubs, and get involved in volunteer work. In essence, you need to make yourself stand out from the rest of the pack. Also important are letters of recommendation, interviews, and the essay, which is especially important when applying to very select schools.

Q. Do SAT prep courses really help improve SAT scores?

A. According to the latest research, the only effective prep courses are the math review courses. Findings show that math skills like algebra and geometry can be learned or re-learned through intensive study, whereas verbal and reading skills have to be acquired over a longer period of time. Improving math skills is often a matter of practicing problem solving and learning techniques that increase speed and accuracy. To improve reading skills, you need to read various types of articles covering a wide range of topics so that you become accustomed to seeing completely different topics on the same test.

Q. What are interviewers looking for when interviewing a student?

A. Different interviewers look for different qualities, but there are five basic areas that all good colleges focus on when conducting any interview. They are:

- Intellectual Potential: Be prepared to answer questions about your high school courses, favorite books, news events, or anything else that might show intellectual promise. Several days before the interview, look through several newspapers and become familiar with current events. If an opportunity arises for you to mention something in the news, you'll earn points for being well versed.

- Motivation: Make a list of your accomplishments before the interview and make sure you can talk about them in a way that will demonstrate your drive to be successful. As you list your accomplishments, awards, achievements, etc., be prepared to explain why these were important or significant.

- Maturity: Be sure to maintain a relaxed and confident demeanor throughout the interview. Don't make jokes with the interviewer, but don't be somber, either. The best way to attack an interview is to answer the questions seriously but calmly, always making eye contact with the interviewer. Men should wear a conservative suit while women should wear a dress or suit. Remember, first impressions can mean a lot and may even set the mood for the rest of the interview.

- Leadership: Good schools that receive many applications from excellent students are looking for those intangible qualities that set individuals apart. Leadership is one of those qualities that "all" schools are after. When you participate in extracurricular activities, always strive for leadership roles. When talking about your activities, make sure you emphasize how well you've carried out your responsibilities and leadership roles and how well these have helped prepare you for college.

- Overall Image: This is one of those intangible qualities that is determined by what the interviewer thinks of you as a person. Image may depend on your personality, ability to respond to questions, body language, honesty and frankness, confidence and poise, and articulateness. It's a good idea to go through mock interviews in order to get feedback on speech problems, annoying habits or anything else that might interfere with a smooth interview performance.

High School 4-Year Timetable

A common mistake high school students make is waiting until their junior or senior year before making serious plans for college. Getting into the college of your choice requires that you begin early in your high school years, preferably in the 9th grade. It's a whole lot easier to start off right and stay on track than it is to start slowly and have to catch up.

The following is a 4-year timetable that outlines the kinds of things you need to be doing or thinking about throughout your four years of high school. Use this timetable as guide after consulting with your school guidance counselor.

Freshman Year

1. Start off on the right track by developing good study habits and sticking with them. There's no substitute for good grades when applying to college.

2. Study the academic requirements of select colleges and plan your academic schedule to meet the toughest requirements you can find. When it comes to college admissions, it's better to be overqualified.

3. Become involved in no more than two school activities. It's to your advantage to be committed to your activities and to strive for leadership roles rather than spread yourself out too thin and not do any of them well.

Sophomore Year

1. Sign up for the toughest courses you can take and study hard to get good grades.

2. Commit to no more than "one" school or community activity. Your sophomore year should be dedicated to achieving high grades and taking tough courses, which will then set you up for your third and fourth years of high school.

3. Continue looking at college programs and begin deciding on some college choices.

Junior Year

1. Make a tentative list of your top ten college choices and make sure your academic requirements meet theirs. Take any additional coursework if necessary.

2. Write to colleges to get information about scholarships, financial aid packages and specific programs in which you're interested.

3. Prepare for and take the SAT and/or ACT. Allow yourself enough time to study properly.

4. Become involved in both school and community service. Again, always aim for leadership roles, since leadership is the prime quality good colleges are looking for.

Senior Year

1. If possible, retake the SAT or ACT. Since the highest score counts, it won't hurt to try again.

2. Send away for application forms from the colleges of your choice. When filling them out, be neat and very careful. When writing an essay, do several drafts and then have someone with good editing skills check it over for spelling, grammar, punctuation, etc. Many colleges consider the essay as important as SAT scores.

3. Submit your application as early as possible. Like all other committees, admissions committees get pressed for time and may not be as careful with late applications as they are with earlier ones. Sending your in early will ensure that it gets the full attention it deserves. If you don't get letters within three weeks confirming that the colleges have received your applications, call them and make sure they had.

Many high school students begin college not knowing what to expect and being ill-prepared for college level courses. Don't be one of those students. By starting now, your road through the early years of college - the time most premedical students drop out or are weeded out - will be far easier and much more rewarding. Precollege preparation will give you a definite advantage over students who'll be overwhelmed by new information and who have never learned how to study properly. The next chapter outlines techniques and strategies for studying, learning, memorizing and test-taking for both high school and college students.

3

Study, Learning & Test Taking Skills

Some students are "naturals" at study. They catch on, learn quickly and remember facts easily. Some don't do as well because they have trouble paying attention or because they've never developed the kinds of study and learning skills their successful classmates have. The difference in performance is not so much a matter of IQ. than it is of behavior and attitude. Research has clearly shown that these two qualities can have a tremendous effect on success in the class room.

Successful students "behave" in certain ways that ensure success. They have the right attitude, they're motivated, they pay attention, they're more relaxed, and they ignore distractions that interfere with learning. And when they need help with school work, they know how to get it. None of these things is inborn, but they can be learned.

Studies have identified four areas that will help an individual become a better all around student. They sound simple because they are. But they will help you achieve success whether you're a high school student or a college senior. They are:

- *Paying Attention*
- *Learning and Remembering*
- *Studying*
- *Test-Taking*

How To Pay Attention

For many students, the greatest challenge of the school day is to keep their minds from wandering over every topic except the one being discussed in class. It certainly was a challenge for me. But there are some easy techniques for learning to pay attention.

1. Use self-talk and positive images. If you've ever watched a sporting event, you'll no doubt have noticed that the players often talk to themselves. They use words or sentences to help control attention. Just as we use words to give directions to others, we can use them to direct our own actions as well. Use words or phrases to help you focus. Tell yourself to keep your eyes on the blackboard while the instructor is writing on it to explain a problem. Practice positive self-talk at home in various situations; when playing a game, helping around the house or working at a hobby.

2. Stop negative self-talk. Many students talk to themselves when they're studying or listening to a lecture, but the self-talk is negative and, therefore, not helping them focus on their work. Negative self-talk can lead to a negative attitude about school and about one's self. Don't say things like "It's hopeless. I just can't concentrate on this stuff." Instead, be positive, saying something like, "I can do this. I'm going to listen to everything the teacher is saying." This kind of positive reinforcement feeds on itself and will improve your overall attitude about yourself and your abilities to learn.

3. Stop negative images. Just like negative self-talk, negative or distracting images work against you. You can and must see yourself doing well in school. Picture yourself answering questions correctly in class and feeling good about knowing the answers.

4. Ask questions. Asking questions really helps focus your attention while listening to a lecture or while studying. For example, when reading about World War II, you might ask yourself, "Which countries were our friends and allies? Which were Germany's? Which countries did Germany occupy?" As you're reading, you may also ask, "What's this paragraph saying? Who did what and why? Is the main point true or false?" Asking questions serves two purposes: It will help you bring your wandering mind back to the task at hand, and it will help you remember what you're reading because you're being proactive rather than passive.

5. Set specific study goals. You can set specific goals that will help your attention. Study a lesson until you can explain the main point . . . or solve a specific math problem . . . or know specific names, dates and places mentioned in the text. Remember that many small goals, one after another, are much better and more effective than a single large one.

Developing and Improving Learning and Study Skills

During your school years, you're going to be presented with a large number of new facts, ideas and concepts. How well you learn them is determined not only by natural intelligence but also by the methods or strategies you employ to master all that information. One of the most important aspects of learning is that the information must be understood to be remembered. Plodding through words on a page or memorizing hundreds of facts that seem unrelated is an ineffective way to learn.

Understanding concepts is not something that just happens. It takes work. It requires taking an active interest in the topic, and it requires the ability to relate new information to that already known. This process is called active or "generative" learning, learning that brings interest and knowledge to the task rather than sitting back and expecting the teacher or textbook to do all the work.

In order to develop and improve learning skills, you must first learn how to organize material and how to study effectively. It doesn't matter how bad a teacher may be, it's your responsibility to get the most from your classes through proper note-taking, efficient study habits and good learning techniques. Just as other skills can be honed with practice, the process of gathering information, organizing it, and repeating it during exams can also be honed. The ideal learning process for most students can be diagrammed in this manner:

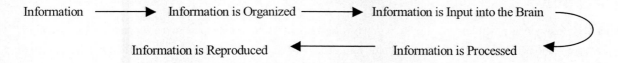

Information is seen and/or heard, organized by note-taking, input into the brain through reading and rewriting, processed and learned through brain conditioning, and reproduced through proper recall. Let's take each stage and see how you can use simple techniques to become a much better student, make exam-taking a lot easier, and get top grades as a result.

A. Organizing Information

The first step in improving learning skills is learning to organize all the information given to you. You do this by note-taking, which is the process of writing down specific information in a way that will be easy to understand and which contains key ideas and words important to the topic in general. Many students never learn to take good notes. They go through high school and college frustrated at having to work so hard and not doing as well as they're capable of doing. Taking good notes makes classes much easier and more interesting because you'll learn the material much faster and with more comprehension. Here are some note-taking strategies:

- Always look over the material to be lectured on beforehand. By knowing something about the topic and being familiar with the information, you'll be able to recognize key ideas and words more readily when you hear them. There's nothing more frustrating than being so unfamiliar with what's being said that you can't even concentrate on the lecture. Even if can't read the material beforehand, at least skim through it to get the main ideas. Most textbooks provide "maps" such as the introduction, headings and summaries that will help you find your way through the subject matter.

- As you begin taking notes, don't write everything down word for word. This is a waste of time and will keep you from paying attention to the important ideas in the lecture. Instead, listen for key ideas and write them down, along with important facts, dates and other information pertinent to those key ideas. Later on, you can fill in any missing pieces from your text or other sources. The outline of your notes should look something like this:

Title of Topic
> A. *Main idea or concept*
>> 1. Pertinent information about idea
>>> a. key point
>>> b. key point
>> 2. Pertinent information about idea
>
> B. *Second main idea or concept*
>> 1. Pertinent information about idea
>>> a. key point
>>> b. key point
>>> c. key point
>> 2. Pertinent information about idea
>>> a. key point
>>> b. key point
>
> C. *Third main idea or concept*

- After class (as soon as possible), you should sit down with your notes and rewrite them in a clear and organized manner. If there are sections that don't make sense, or some important gaps that need to be filled, use your text or other source to clear up any discrepancies and fill in missing information. This is also the time to eliminate clutter that will confuse you when studying for exams. The physical act of reading and rewriting your notes after class reinforces what you hear in lecture and is an excellent way to initiate learning while the material is still fresh in your mind.

- If there are certain facts you absolutely must memorize, such as formulas, equations, definitions, etc., write them out on index cards then use as flash cards for review. Every few days, go through your prepared flash cards until you have the material memorized. Change the order of the cards each time by shuffling them. Also learn the material in reverse. That is, if you're learning the definition of a word, don't only look at the word and learn the definition, look at the definition and be able to identify the word.

B. Inputting Information: The Art of Studying

The second step in improving learning skills is being able to take the material you've organized and inputting it into your brain in the most effective way possible. This takes more effort than organizing information, but once mastered will give you the tools needed to retrieve anything you're given in class. It's a fact that up to 95 percent of the most important textbook information can be located very quickly since only 25 percent of all the written material in a text is really needed. By reading effectively, you can save a tremendous amount of time and energy.

When you study, do some planning ahead of time. A lot of wasted effort goes into studying because students simply don't know the methods that will ensure success. Fact is, the amount of time spent studying is not as important as the way the time is spent. Even two hours of effective study is better than six hours of poor study. And you'll still have four hours left for other important assignments and activities.

One of the biggest complaints I hear from students is that there's never enough time to do all their work. Nonsense. Anyone can develop good study and learning skills if they're really serious about doing well in school. Here are some ways to do that.

- Find your best study time. Different students function differently during various times of the day because we all have unique biological clocks. You need to discover whether you're a morning, afternoon or evening person. Anyone can train themselves to study at just about any time, but you should discover when your "peak" attention and concentration time is. Unless you establish your own right time, you may be wasting as much as 25 percent of your study efforts. You also need to set aside specific times for chores, work and fun on a weekly basis. These schedules should be flexible enough to allow trade-offs and shifts when necessary

- Manage your time efficiently. Part of being a good student is being a good time manager. Stick to your optimal time for the most efficient studying, and try to establish a study routine. Your brain, just like any other organ in your body, will get conditioned to a daily routine and begin preparing for it each day. Never study more than 45 minutes to an hour without taking a 5 to 10 minute break, since studies show that the average student will lose his or her concentration beyond that point.

- Establish a place to study. Whether you live in a one bedroom apartment or a sprawling mansion, you have to set aside your own study area. It can be a desk or a kitchen table, but it must be fairly quiet and have a good light.

- Preview any material before you actually get down to serious studying. Always begin an assignment by previewing the material. Reading the introduction to a chapter, for example, the heading, or the summary. This is like looking at a road map and creating a "mental map" of what's ahead in the assignment. Ask yourself questions as you read. "What conclusions can I draw from this? What are the main ideas? What is the author trying to tell me?"

- As you rewrite your notes, say the material out loud to yourself. The combined physical acts of writing and speaking are an excellent mental exercise and will improve recall of the material almost immediately. Also, as you rewrite your notes, test yourself on the material. You can make up questions pertaining to the topic and answer them.

- Form a study group and exchange ideas with other students. Being actively involved by discussing the week's material with other students will force you to concentrate on the material and help you absorb it much better.

C. Processing Information: Recall and Memorization

The third step in improving study skills and perhaps the most important in terms of helping you prepare for exams is conditioning the brain to recall information. Conditioning your brain to repeat the material you've organized is a matter of not waiting till the last minute. The key to conditioning any part of the body, including the brain, is time and repetition.

Some memory experts have suggested that we never really forget what we learn. Everything we input into our brain is somehow stored there indefinitely, much like data is stored on a computer disk. What we call poor memory is really an inability to retrieve that data. Here are some ways to help you strengthen and develop memory and to increase your ability to process the information you input.

- Make a conscious decision to remember. This very simple and obvious point is the first step in effective recall. Tell yourself that you plan to remember! Before the lecture begins, say to yourself, "I'm going to remember what's being said today." Most students go into a lecture assuming they're not going to remember the material and, therefore, they don't use their subconscious to input information.

- At the end of each day, go over the material you've input that day. Psychologists tell us that most forgetting occurs shortly after learning has taken place. A good technique is writing down the main points learned, then spending ten minutes thinking about each point.

- At the end of the week, review the notes you've accumulated since the class first began. This brief review will prevent you from totally forgetting the material and will keep your mind continually thinking about previous information. Try to analyze the material in order to intensify the impression it makes in your mind. Work it over and become involved in it. Ask yourself questions that will force yourself to think about it. If you can, make your own applications, examples and illustrations to reinforce memorization.

- Find the main idea of the topic. Students make the mistake of concentrating on everything rather than trying to find the main idea. As you read your text, ask yourself, "What's the point here?" When you learn the main ideas and principles, the remaining information will all fit into place.

- Use the flash cards you've made as often as it tales to learn things you need to memorize. Remember to rearrange the cards each time and reverse the order of learning so that you can recognize material no matter how it's presented. Go over this material at odd times, not only at a certain time each day.

- A week or so before the exam, begin lecturing to yourself from your notes. While studying, pretend you're the teacher and try to teach as you study. In this way, you'll have two avenues that information can be absorbed into your brain - through your eyes and through your ears. Because your brain will be picking up two separate and different signals, you'll increase your ability to retain any information your brain receives. If there's material that will need to be written out on the exam, practice writing it out as well as saying it. Remember, physical actions coupled with mental actions increase recall by as much as 50 percent.

- Anticipate exam questions. By thinking up exam questions from important ideas, concepts, words, etc., you'll improve the quality of your study by thinking about the material in more depth. You'll also be pleasantly surprised when you see the same questions on the exam.

- Discuss the information to be learned with others. Not only will discussion of the material reinforce it in your mind, hearing it from others will increase its processing in your mind.

- Use mental techniques or tricks to help you remember names, definitions, words, etc. that are giving you problems. A technique called "mental imaging" can help you memorize anything with a little practice. All you need to do is associate the word or principle to be memorized with any mental image that will help you make the association between the two. Close your eyes and form a picture of the image in your mind's eye. Another device called mnemonics uses a word composed of the first letters of the item to be memorized. For example, ROY G BIV is the mnemonic for the visible light spectrum of red, orange, yellow, green, blue, indigo and violet.

D. Reproducing Information

The final step, and the one you ultimately work toward, is being able to take the information you've processed and reproduce it on an exam. If you've studied effectively and haven't crammed, you should have little trouble with this stage. However, here are some ways that will make reproducing information easier.

- Never study the night before the exam. Even if you don't fell completely confident about the material, try to relax. If you think you really need to look over your notes just one more time, then briefly skim through them before bed, then forget about them. Your subconscious mind will go over the material as you sleep.

- If the exam includes questions that will require knowledge of formulas or equations, here's a technique that works for students who freeze during those kinds of exams. As soon as you get your exam paper, turn it over and write down the formulas or equations you'll need before looking at any of the questions. In this way, you won't get flustered into forgetting information when you begin reading the exam. It'll be right on the back of the paper whenever you need it.

- Whenever possible, answer the question before looking at the alternatives. This technique helps avoid confusion when there are several similar answers

- Watch for restrictive words. Words like most, only, rarely, immediate, primarily, etc., or any number such as first, fifth, etc. are sometimes a clue that the answer is wrong.

- Look for negative and all inclusive words. Words such as never, not at all, at no time, not ever, nothing, all, always, entirely and without exception usually indicate a false statement.

- Look for qualifying words. Words such as generally, usually, and frequently often indicate a true statement.

- Unless you're penalized for guessing wrong answers, always make a guess. The rule here is to eliminate as many obviously wrong answers as possible in order to increase your odds of choosing the right answer. When guessing, there are certain clues to look for in order to increase the chances of your guessing correctly. These are:

  1. A long alternative is usually more correct that a short one.
  2. The more general alternative is often more correct than the specific one.
  3. When two alternatives have slight differences between them, one is likely to be correct. Eliminate all other answers and choose between these two.
  4. When two totally opposite options are give, one of them is likely to be correct. Eliminate all other answers and choose between these two.
  5. When the alternative are all numerical, the correct answer is not likely to be one of the numerical extremes.
  6. Look for grammatical correctness. Questions that end with "an" often indicate that the answer begins with a vowel. Questions ending with "a" will have an answer beginning with a consonant.

- As soon as you get to a question that seems too difficult to answer, go on to the next one immediately. Don't become anxious or annoyed because you don't think you can answer a question - your subconscious mind will automatically begin work on the information even as you answer other questions. Soon, the answer to that seemingly impossible question will just pop into your mind automatically.

- After you finish the exam, go back and reread your answers, changing and adding as needed. Don't rush out of the exam as soon as you're done. Take your time and edit your work carefully.

Overcoming Test Anxiety

It's good to be concerned about taking a test. It's not good to get "test anxiety." This excessive worry about doing well on an exam can mean disaster for a student. Students who suffer from test anxiety tend to worry about success in school, especially doing well on exams. They worry about their future and can extremely self-critical. Instead of feeling challenged by the prospect of success, they become afraid of failure. This makes them anxious about tests and about their own abilities in general. Ultimately, they become so worked up that they feel incompetent about the subject matter.

One of the biggest problems with test anxiety is that it can direct one's attention away from the material to be learned and away from productive ways to study. Your thoughts may turn to self-criticism, to blaming teachers for your predicament, and to worry over what others will think. As a result, you'll become less organized and less effective in your study habits, which then leads to poor test scores and low grades. Some students even decide that poor grades are a sure sign they're not smart enough to do well. This leads to frustration and even worse study habits and test scores. It's a viscous cycle, but there are ways to reduce to this anxiety. Here are some tips:

- Space out your studying over days or weeks and review it more than once. By doing this, you should feel prepared at exam time. Never cram the night before, since this only increases anxiety and interferes with clear thinking. Leave your learning alone. Your brain will remain active, sorting and reworking the material you've input over the last several weeks. Then get a good night's sleep. Rest, exercise and eating well are as important to test-taking as they are to other schoolwork.

- Try to maintain a regular routine during exam week so that you can concentrate on schoolwork and, at the same time, remain calm and relaxed. Nothing is more disruptive to good study habits and effective learning than to start something new during exam week that is going to take away from your goals.

- Stay away from students who panic before an exam. Panic is contagious and can be spread to even the best student. Students who have negative attitudes will invariably rub some of those attitudes off on others.

- Come prepared by packing a special exam kit, which includes pens, pencils, erasers, paper, ruler, calculator, Kleenex, and perhaps a small snack you can quietly much on.

- Read the directions carefully when the test is handed out. If you don't understand something, ask for an explanation right away. Don't wait until you're well into the exam.

- Look quickly at the entire exam to see what types of questions are included (multiple choice, matching, essay, true/false) and, if possible, the number of points each is worth. This will help you pace yourself. Always allow more time for sections worth more points, but don't spend so much time that you'll miss everything else. The important thing is to budget your time wisely so that you can most effectively complete the exam.

- When answering essay questions, answer the easiest questions first. This will get you going and prevent you from thinking too much about not knowing information. Write short, snappy sentences that say something. Avoid extra words that will take up time, and always try to be brief, concise and accurate. Read the instructions and watch for words such as list, discuss, explain, etc. I take off quite a few points when students are asked to "discuss" or "explain" but only list or give a short, few word answer. Write the essay exactly as the instructions call for.

- Admit to yourself that you're not going to know every answer. Instead of saying "I'm not going to do well," say "I'll know most of the answers, but there are going to be some that I probably won't know." In this way, you won't be shocked when you come across a question you can't answer. You'll simply go on to questions you can answer while your subconscious mind works on the ones you couldn't get right away. Before long, if you've studied well, answers will begin to pop into your head and you'll begin flying through the exam.

You may seem uncomfortable with these approaches to learning and studying, but that's natural with any new way of doing things. After you've used these techniques for a while, though, they'll become as natural as the study methods you're using now and much more rewarding and effective.

4

The Premedical Curriculum

Beginning Your Premed Strategy

Ideally, premedical planning should begin during the later years of high school or early years of college. Realistically, not many students have these kinds of ambitions until they've become acquainted with various career options. This usually occurs by the second or third year of college when courses taken channel particular interests in a certain direction. If you're a late bloomer, or just someone who hadn't made a firm commitment to medical school until now, don't worry; the days when medical schools preferred only science majors are long gone. Some schools, like some businesses, even prefer to have individuals they can mold into their own way of thinking and who haven't developed biases or bad habits during their undergraduate years.

Be wary of majoring in "Premed." Some schools actually look unfavorably on this major and are considering eliminating it altogether because they feel that it's too narrow a preparation for medical school. Medical schools realize that a student needs to have an alternate career should he or she fail to gain admission to a medical school. So, as long as you complete all the required coursework needed for admission, you should major in anything you like and would enjoy doing in case medical schools reject you.

A high percentage of non-science majors are very successful in getting accepted each year. In fact, over the years, it has been shown time and again that non-science majors do just as well as science majors. If you do major in anything other than science, you can use this to your advantage by showing admissions committees that you're mature enough to consider other career options but are still sincere enough about medical school to complete all the necessary science coursework.

A recent study looking at four types of college major clearly demonstrated no significant differences in scores on any MCAT subtest, except for the reading part. Physical science majors obtained the lowest scores in that area. One of the more interesting things found in the study was that social science and humanities majors took as little as 40 percent of their credits in science courses compared to 56 percent taken by physical science majors, yet both groups had similar academic performances. In other words, you don't have to give up courses you'd like to take because you think that taking some extra science classes will help you. They really don't.

A more important, but not surprising, fact was that on the empathy test (designed to rate interpersonal aspects of the doctor-patient relationship, physical science majors scored the lowest while social science majors scored the highest. In light of this, more and more attention is being given to attitudes and personal qualities among different categories of undergraduate programs because a student's non-science major may reveal more about his or her ability as a future doctor than previously believed. After all, once many of the details regarding organic chemistry and other physical sciences are long forgotten, attitudes, sensitivity to interpersonal issues and ability to develop good doctor-patient relationships are really the critical factors in health care.

So, now that you know a science major is definitely not a prerequisite for admission to medical school, you need to know the requirements that are. You also need to know the kinds of courses medical schools looks favorably on and the ones that some medical faculty members have told me can enhance a student's overall credentials.

Required Courses For Admission

Of course, the kind of coursework required varies from school to school, but almost all medical schools insist that you have certain courses they feel will prepare you for their curriculums. These are:

Biology (with laboratory)	1 year
Inorganic Chemistry (with laboratory)	1 year
Organic Chemistry (with laboratory)	1 year
General Physics (with laboratory)	1 year
English	1 year

In addition to these basic requirements, quite a few medical schools also require:

Mathematics (through calculus)	1 year
Behavioral/Social Sciences	1 year
Humanities	1 year

Medical schools would like their students to become "total physicians," capable of understanding human needs as well as diagnosing disease; able to communicate and respond effectively and compassionately. A curriculum that demonstrates a desire to enhance your ability to deal with other human beings looks more favorable than one filled with nothing but science courses.

According to Dr. Pellegrino, writing in the *Journal of the American Medical Association*, "The central act of medicine - making a clinical decision - is only part scientific. To make a right and good decision for a particular patient requires thinking more properly derived from the liberal arts and humanities." And the conclusion of a Rockefeller Foundation-sponsored conference on liberal arts and premedical education was that overemphasizing technical expertise has harmful effects on pre-med and medical education. These effects are alleviated by encouraging a more broadly based undergraduate curriculum.

Your electives should not only include recommended science courses but should also include a wide range of humanities, behavioral and social science courses that will give admissions committee members an indication of your sincere desire to become a well-rounded individual. Nothing destroys a doctor-patient relationship faster than a doctor's inability to relate to his or her patient. Medical schools recognize the importance of personal attributes and look for individuals they feel will be both physician and humanitarian.

Recommended Courses for Admission

Naturally, you won't be able to take every course you would like at your college or university. Be selective in your choices and consider taking those courses that will add dimension to your character. These may or may not be science courses, but they should be courses that can be applied to the study of medicine. The following are courses many schools recommend but don't necessarily require. An asterisk preceding the name of the course indicates that at least 20 medical schools strongly recommend it.

* Biochemistry	Computer Science
* Calculus	Psychology
* Embryology	Sociology
* Genetics	Anatomy
* Physical Chemistry	Histology
* Statistics	Foreign Language

Some Valuable Non-Science Courses

Here also are some humanities, social science, and behavioral science courses that will look favorable on your transcript.

Anthropology	Music
Art / Art History	Philosophy
History	Psychology
Literature	Sociology

Don't neglect these courses just because you feel that you'll never use them in the medical profession. The "well-rounded" physician (most medical school faculty members are) will certainly be conversant with many of these subjects. It would be to your advantage to introduce yourself to as many humanities subjects as you can in order to begin your development as a potential physician.

Although science is an essential ingredient of a broad education, studies in the social sciences and humanities are equally important for a thorough understanding of contemporary society. Physicians must draw upon history, economics, politics, philosophy and the culture of people in order to appreciate the many dimensions of human behavior and human problems. Physicians cannot be narrow-minded individuals and effectively solve the problems of the sick in our society. Premedical education must prepare you to understand both the scientific and the personal side of human suffering. To do this, you need to develop a curriculum that will blend the sciences and humanities so that you can increase your awareness of community, societal, cultural and global issues in an increasingly complex world. This concept of being both healer and humanitarian is so important that the American Board of Internal Medicine has recently added a new requirement to its certification process. Each new applicant taking the specialty examination in Internal Medicine must be certified by the director of his/her residency program as demonstrating "humanistic" qualities. As a premedical student, then, it would serve you well to take several extra humanities classes throughout your undergraduate career.

Premedical students often lack the opportunity (usually because they take a lot of science courses) to develop good writing skills. Since physicians need to acquire skills in writing and persuasive reasoning, you would do well to take more writing courses. An added incentive: The MCAT's essay section identifies poor writing skills. Therefore, develop the art of skillful writing by taking classes that make you write. You won't regret it, even if you never go on to medical school. One of the most important criteria many corporate officers have for hiring a person is good communications skills, both oral and written. Several have even told me they place greater value on these than grades. Here are samples of typical premedical curriculums offered at selective and highly distinguished undergraduate schools:

School A

Freshman Year	General Chemistry (with lab), 15 quarter hours
	Analytic Geometry and Calculus, 15 quarter hours
	English Composition, 9 quarter hours
	World History, 9 quarter hours
	Electives, 3 quarter hours

Sophomore Year	General Biology (with lab) / Cell Biology (with lab), 16 quarter hours
	Organic Chemistry (with lab), 15 quarter hours
	Introductory Physics (with lab) / Modern Physics, 12 quarter hours
	Literature, 9 quarter hours
	Electives, 3 quarter hours

Junior/Senior Years	English Composition	Psychology
	Political Science	Sociology

Zoology   Philosophy

Other requirements

School B

Freshman Year   General Biology (with lab), 8 semester hours

General Chemistry (with lab), 8 semester hours

College Writing, 6 semester hours

Finite Mathematics / Calculus, 7 semester hours

Biology Elective, 3 semester hours

Sophomore Year   Cell Biology / Developmental Biology, 9 semester hours

Organic Chemistry (with lab), 8 semester hours

College Physics (with lab), 10 semester hours

Biology Electives, 6 semester hours

Junior/Senior Years   Genetics

Electives and other requirements

School B strongly recommends that students take all the required science courses during the first three years of study in order to prepare for the MCAT or DAT. The closer together the core material is taken, the more organized the student can be in taking the MCAT. Furthermore, School B emphasizes that medical schools take note of the sequence and timing of the courses taken in a premed program. They look skeptically at programs that delay important courses such as physics and organic chemistry until the junior or senior year.

Overall Academic Characteristics

If there's one important academic characteristic that medical schools are searching for in their applicants, it's a broad educational base. Science, naturally, is important in the study of medicine. Humanities (art, music, literature) are important in developing a more cultured and diverse background. Skills in communication (both oral and written) are without question one of the most criteria in the selection process because they are critical in a physician's ability to interrelate with others. Behavioral sciences are vital in developing a physician's awareness of human personality and the needs of the community as well as society.

In essence, your undergraduate curriculum must not only show that you're interested in science but that you also seek to expand your cultural base and broaden your horizons. Intellect is only part of being a physician. You must understand that society places a physician in high regard and, therefore, medical schools accept applicants they feel will represent their schools and their profession in the highest tradition. According to the president of a major university, medicine is so diverse that it can benefit from all kinds of backgrounds and interests. To give you an idea of how much this kind of philosophy is being accepted, the Association of American Medical Colleges has made the following five recommendations with regard to medical school admissions policies:

1. All college and university students should be required to study broadly the natural and social sciences and the humanities.

2. Medical school faculties should require only "essential" courses and should stop recommending additional courses beyond these.

3. College faculties should make scholarly endeavor and the development of effective writing skills integral features of undergraduate education.

4. Medical schools should use admissions criteria that appraise independent learning, analytic skills, and the development of attitudes and values essential for those in a caring profession who are to contribute to the welfare of society.

5. Communication between college and medical school faculty concerning admission criteria should be improved.

These premedical guidelines have been established because, in order to understand and have sympathy for those who seek help, the medical association feels that a physician must be deeply attentive to varieties of human behavior, experiences and personalities. Being a non-physician, therefore, is just as important at times as being a physician. Students selected as future doctors must exhibit maturity, intelligence and understanding.

An excellent way to gauge how successful premedical programs are is to find out how practicing physicians feel about their college educations. A recent survey was conducted in which participating physicians were asked how they felt about the emphasis placed on premedical science and non-science courses and, based on their experiences and current perspectives, which areas they thought needed more emphasis. An overwhelming 72 percent said that more emphasis should have been placed on non-science courses in college, especially humanities such as English, literature and philosophy. One physician thought that the chemistry and physics proved useless, another said that the humanities were the best preparation for the practice of medicine, and others urged students to do intensive study in literature and the arts. This survey of physicians clearly demonstrated something lacking in premedical education.

Once a student enters medical school and goes on to a residency position, the opportunities for a broad liberal education dwindle away. After the rigors of medical training, many physicians suddenly find that something is missing in their educational background. By then, they feel it's too late to correct the weaknesses because the demands of a doctor's life leave little room to go back and try to add the missing pieces. The lesson here is that, although science is important in the medical school admissions process, you should look ahead and prepare yourself for life beyond medical school. According to many doctors, humanities is one of the most important ways to do that.

Getting a Head Start on Coursework

The Medical School Admission Requirements Handbook (which every medical school advisor at your college will have) will give you a good idea of what certain medical schools expect in general and what a few expect in addition. In this way you can begin taking required courses early and also give yourself enough flexibility to take some additional courses to build your credentials. Taking required courses early and then taking additional courses later on serves three purposes.

1. You can take the MCAT in the spring of your junior year and will have had all the coursework that's covered on the exam. This gives you enough time for preparing and reviewing. Statistics show that juniors perform best on the MCAT because the test material is still familiar to them.

2. Any additional coursework you take will not only build your credentials but may help you perform better on the MCAT. Advanced courses naturally build on introductory courses and force you to review concepts you may have forgotten or never quite understood the first time.

3. Medical school curricula are rigorous. It would be to your advantage to take some advanced courses in biology and chemistry in order to prepare yourself for the avalanche of information you'll be exposed to as a first year medical student. I've spoken to a few medical students who've taken advance courses such as biochemistry, genetics, histology and advanced physiology before entering medical school and they've all told me that it was extremely helpful to have had them.

Premedical Syndrome

An increasing number of medical schools are becoming concerned about a growing condition called "premed syndrome." It begins early in a student's undergraduate career and gets progressively worse by the third year of college. I've seen it first hand as a student, then as a teaching assistant and a faculty member. It seems that the drive for medical school admission and the competition for high grades becomes so intense that premedical students develop an attitude totally opposite to what's considered important to becoming a good doctor.

According to many advisors, faculty and fellow students, premedical students are seen as excessively competitive, overly grade-conscious, narrow in interests, less sociable, aggressive and more interested in money or prestige. Many premeds become so narrow in scope that they plan their entire second and third years around the MCAT and the admissions process. They alter study habits, lighten course loads, refrain from taking any class that would risk lowering their GPA, withdraw from extracurricular activities (a mistake!) and pass up work opportunities. I've known premedical students who passed up or dropped out of great courses because they couldn't afford to get anything less than an A. In essence, they gave up a wonderful and crucial part of their education just to do well on one exam.

Premedical students often take one science course after another, as if they believe that this is the best ticket into medical school. They overcommit themselves to science for the sake of the MCAT rather than pursuing courses which would make them better doctors. Some medical schools, unfortunately, still look for aggressive type students because these kinds of students are usually highly motivated and do well under pressure. However, many more medical schools are beginning to look at premed syndrome qualities as negative characteristics and, instead, are leaning toward more broad-minded and people-oriented candidates.

Because liberal arts majors have proven over the years to be just as successful in medical school as science majors, admissions committees are more inclined to look at a student's overall personality characteristics than at his or her performance in a glut of science courses. In fact, one study has shown that English majors performed as well in medical school as chemistry majors. Therefore, to avoid being tagged with the premed syndrome label, don't waste your first three years of college. Enjoy what a college education has to offer and, without giving up anything for science, become well-rounded. This is now the trend for admissions decisions and policies.

Grades

GPA is perhaps the single most important factor in determining success for admission. Although medical schools weigh many factors in their selection process, and some schools say that no one individual factor is weighed more than any other, by and large grades are definitely important. This is the case for several reasons. One, your grades are the only way to really quantify performance against others in your class. And two, your GPA is seen as a reflection of your work ethic. When I look at a student's GPA, for example, I never think of it as a measure of intelligence but rather as the ability of the student to work hard. After all, how many bright students get poor grades because they won't study and how many not so bright students get As and Bs because they work much harder than their counterparts?

If you look at the grades of students who have been successful in gaining admission during the past few years, only about 5 percent of those with C averages were able to get into medical school. Your chances, therefore, improve dramatically as your grades go up. Grades can also have a dampening effect on lower-than-average MCAT scores. If your MCAT scores are not very good, but your GPA is fairly high, it could mean the difference between an interview or not.

In most years, the average GPA for incoming medical students has been between 3.4 and 3.6, which demonstrates the importance grades make in the selection process. But despite emphasis on grades, premedical GPAs have decreased during the past decade. The last three students I helped gain admission to medical school have all had GPAs less than 3.0. One, in fact, had a GPA of 2.5! She's now an M.D. in a residency program and doing very well. Obviously there were other factors we worked on which helped these students overcome low grades. I'll discuss those in later chapters.

Studies show that four year graduation and dropout rates are almost identical for students with undergraduate GPAs between 3.0 and 4.0. It's only for those few students with GPAs below 3.0 that dropout rates begin to increase. Therefore, admissions committees usually use 3.0 as an unofficial threshold for determining success in medical school, since they expect 97 percent of students with that kind of GPA to graduate from medical programs.

In general, you need to maintain a high GPA and, at the same time, remember that you shouldn't let your grades get in the way of your education. In other words, show the admissions committee members that you've gotten more out of your four years of college than a 3.5 GPA. As I've mentioned before, medical schools have no place for someone who has done little else but think about grades. In the next chapter, I discuss ways in which many of the students I've spoken to have turned their non-academic activities and spare time into productive strategies for success.

There's one other factor about grades that I feel is important. Don't be dismayed if most of the schools you read about have incoming students with GPAs of 3.6 or higher. Keep in mind that the range is often very great. The students I helped get in prove that point. Admissions committees take many factors into consideration when selecting students, and GPA is only one of them. There are a few schools that expect applicants to have a minimum GPA in order to be considered any further, but the majority of schools realize that extraordinary circumstances occur than can prevent an individual from doing as well as he or she could (working while going to school, for example).

The rule of thumb seems to be that too many Cs hurt, Bs don't hurt but can help, and As definitely help. I'm not sure how hard and fast that is, but you can be certain that the closer your GPA is to 3.5, the better your odds for admission become. The purpose of the next few chapter is to give you that extra edge that could mean the difference between admission and rejection. Study them carefully and begin your strategy for success.

5

The Application & Admissions Process

The process of medical school application and admission has been changing over the years partly because of changes in the number of medical school applicants. As an example, in 1997-98, almost 47,000 applicants applied to medical schools compared to 17,000 in 1987-88 and only 9,500 in 1967-68. The selection process has also gone through significant changes, especially during the past decade. Despite the changes, and despite the total number of applicants, every medical school has maintained its own particular strategy for identifying and selecting what they hope is their "ideal" medical student. The guidelines in this chapter are followed by most medical school admissions committees, and they should help you understand the overall admissions process.

Where to Begin

You should begin by obtaining the most recent issue of the *Medical School Admission Requirements* published by the AAMC. This book doesn't go into a great deal of detail about particular medical school programs, but it's an excellent source of general information regarding the application process and should be an indispensable guide for anyone seriously considering medical school.

The rule is, apply one year before the date that you would be starting medical school. So, if you're a junior, you would apply during the summer or fall of your junior year and, if accepted, would begin medical school the following summer. It's extremely important to pay attention to school application dates and deadlines. Most medical schools begin accepting applications June 15 and usually won't accept any application after their particular deadline (which may be anywhere from November 1st onward depending on the school). In order to meet the deadlines, make sure that you take the MCAT in the spring (preferably) or, at the very latest, in the fall of the year preceding your anticipated entrance. Schools requiring the MCAT will not review your application unless your MCAT scores are available to them for examination. Premedical advisors should guide you through the process.

It's important that you apply as early as you can because the peak time at most medical school admissions offices is September through December. Once applications begin to roll in during September, the entire process slows down and there's always that improbable chance that some part of your application will not get to where it's supposed to get. This rarely happens, but I would recommend getting your application in the mail before September at the latest. And since most schools don't start processing the application forms until all the materials are on file, you can rectify any problems with transcripts, application forms, etcetera in plenty of time for proper evaluation.

American Medical College Admissions Service (AMCAS)

The main responsibility of AMCAS is to ensure that all medical school application materials are complete and correct and to distribute the materials, along with the latest two MCAT scores taken since April, 1991, to as many medical schools as you choose to apply to, provided they participate in this service. For the 1999 entering class, 112 medical schools are participating in this service. All other schools require new applicants and transfer students to contact schools directly for application instructions.

AMCAS is in no way involved in the selection process and is not affiliated with any medical school. Its only function is to act as an intermediary between you the applicant and whichever medical schools you designate on the AMCAS application forms. Application fees and instructions for payment and waivers are included in the application materials.

The AMCAS forms can be quite complicated to the uninitiated student. Therefore, you need to obtain several copies from your premedical advisor as soon as possible in order to begin filling them out. I say several copies because I've yet to see anyone fill one out correctly and neatly on their first attempt. Make sure you fill out a practice form first, then check it thoroughly before typing the final copy to be sent to AMCAS. If your school doesn't have a premedical advisor, you may get AMCAS application materials by writing directly to:

American Medical College Application Service
2501 M Street, NW
Washington, D.C. 20037-1300
(202) 828-0600
E-mail: amcas@aamc.org

Neatness is very important, since the copies that will be distributed to medical schools are a reflection of you. A sloppy AMCAS form with misspellings and grammatical errors can put an admissions committee off and, though in and of itself will not be the deciding factor, can certainly be one of the negative factors in your chances for gaining admission. Remember, a very neat and thorough AMCAS application won't guarantee acceptance, but a sloppy application form with many errors can surely contribute to the rejection of applicants who might be on the borderline.

The concept of AMCAS is very useful since the application procedure saves you the time and effort of sending individual applications to every school you apply to. Your application will be quickly sent back to you if you've made any serious errors, which is another good reason to begin early and apply as soon as you can. Delay is critical in the selection process. But as long as you send the AMCAS application early enough (June 1 is the earliest date), you can still get it returned, corrected, and sent back in plenty of time.

One important note: make sure you arrange to have all your transcripts from all your undergraduate, graduate, and professional schools sent to AMCAS before you send the AMCAS application form to AMCAS. When you obtain the packet containing the AMCAS forms and information, be sure to read the instructions carefully before filling out the application. Send the enclosed transcript request forms to all the colleges, universities, and professional schools you've attended so that they have enough time to send out your transcripts before AMCAS receives all your other application materials.

AMCAS and Initial Screening of Applicants

Many schools use the AMCAS application for initial screening. Students whose applications suggest they would have trouble handling a medical school curriculum, or whose qualifications aren't up to par, are rejected. All other applicants are then sent an additional supplementary application packet with information regarding other requirements such as letters of evaluation, additional fees, etc. These extra items must be sent directly to the medical school and not to AMCAS

Because the AMCAS application is often used for initial screening, it's very important that you make as good an impression as possible. Don't be afraid to emphasize your good qualities, since these will be the selling points that may very well award you an interview. You have nothing to lose by marketing your talents and strengths and everything to gain in terms of successful admission. After all, what good will your efforts and hard work do for you if no one on the admissions committee knows about them? It's like writing a book and not marketing it. It could have been a best seller but instead it sits on the shelf, unread.

Never sell yourself short and, above all, don't underestimate the value an admissions committee member will place on your work or activity. What you might think is insignificant, a medical school may consider highly desirable as far as overall preparation for a medical career. This is especially important if your grades or MCAT scores are not as high as they should be. At the end of this chapter is a filled-out example of an AMCAS application form. Use it as a guide only.

The Autobiographical Sketch

An important part of the AMCAS application is the autobiographical sketch. Here is where intangible factors such as extracurricular activities (discussed in the next chapter) can really stand out and make the admissions committee take notice. This is also the part of the application that could convince a medical school that, regardless of some other shortcomings, you have what it takes to become a good physician.

Take a good deal of time on this part. Don't just write an autobiographical sketch and expect it to be acceptable the first or even the second time around. If professional writers sometimes revise their work a dozen times, surely you can do it at least two or three. Read and reread your sketch several times, making changes and corrections as needed. Put it aside for a few days, then come back to it again with fresh ideas and a better way to phrase sentences. Going back to your work after not seeing it will make editing easier. Mistakes will literally leap off the page at you, and you'll remember things you may not have thought of during the first or second draft.

As you rewrite your sketch, emphasize key accomplishments and, without being too obnoxious, try not to be too modest. Your sketch is one of hundreds and sometimes thousands seen by admissions committees and needs to stand out from the others.

I can't emphasize enough how much this area of the selection process could mean and how you should do everything you can to ensure that, after reading your autobiographical sketch, an admissions committee will be convinced of your potential as a medical student. Your goal here is to clinch that all important interview.

Once you've written several drafts, it's a good idea to have your premed advisor and/or an English major read and edit it for any grammatical errors. A blatant error can make the most understanding committee member have second thoughts. You don't want to ruin an otherwise good application at this point. Here are some items that committee members specifically look for:

- Unique background and life history. Don't dwell on your family background too much unless it's interesting enough to warrant it. Use the bulk of the space allotted on you.

- Unique experiences such as travel abroad, service in the armed forces, etc.

- Unique work experiences such as laboratory research or scientific projects. Always include where you did your volunteer work, as well as when you did it, with whom, exactly what you did, and what your results were. Be concise.

- Publications of any kind are important. If you have an unpublished manuscript, say what the title is and give its status (in preparation, submitted, in press, etc.).

- Volunteer work at a hospital or any organization that served the needs of individuals or the community. Make sure you mention where and when you performed your work and what exactly it was you did. Also state why it was important both to you and the people you helped.

- Statement of future goals, aspiration, and objectives.

Medical schools like to have a diverse student body with varied experiences and unusual backgrounds. Try to convince the admissions committee that you're the kind of individual who will add something special to the incoming freshman class. Without being self-centered, make yourself stand out among the other applicants so that the admissions committee will feel compelled to grant you an interview and find out a little more about you.

Sometimes the decision of whether or not to grant an applicant an interview is based on the contents of his or her autobiographical sketch. If you're a borderline student, make your sketch work for you by giving it all the attention it deserves. Always remember to be specific. Give concrete details. Be serious; never write anything humorous or clever. Your aim is to ensure that the sketch is read with interest when compared with all the others. A friend of mine who interviews many medical school candidates, had the following to say about autobiographical sketches:

"When I read an autobiographical sketch, what I don't want to see is a long exposé about why the student wants to become a doctor. I want to read about his or her accomplishments. After all, a 21 year old has no real experience in medicine, so I don't care to read about medicine. I want to see whether that person is caring, motivated, an independent thinker, and inspires others to act.

Medicine is a very heavy pressure career, and a person who chooses medicine must have demonstrated the ability to make decisions, be independent, and assume a good deal of responsibility. Those are the qualities that need to shine through on the autobiography.

One sketch I remember well was written by a student who was in charge of a school cafeteria. He supervised 60 students and was responsible for scheduling work assignments and vacations, and had to make sure everyone knew what to do during the work day. When I interviewed him several months later, we spent most of the time talking about his work at the cafeteria. I knew from his sketch and the ensuing interview that, even though he didn't have any experience in medicine, he would make a fantastic doctor."

When you're writing your autobiographical sketch, don't make the mistake of thinking that personal accomplishments don't mean much to an admissions committee member. Many times they mean everything. If you've done anything that shows you to be a creative, take-charge, responsible person who leads and inspires others to accomplish goals, include that in your sketch. Any committee member who reads about a person like that would no doubt take notice and say, "Hey, medicine could use someone like that." Look at the sample autobiographical sketch included with the AMCAS form at the end of this chapter. See if you can pick out the points I said were important when writing your sketch.

Non-AMCAS Medical Schools

Medical schools not participating in AMCAS have their own application forms which are to be filled out and sent directly to the medical school or they participate in The University of Texas System Medical and Dental Application Center (UTSMDAC). There's a separate application fee that must be included with your application materials, and the deadlines may or may not be the same as those of AMCAS participating schools. The following is a list of non-AMCAS schools:

Baylor College of Medicine, Houston, TX

Brown University School of Medicine, Providence, RI

Columbia University College of Physicians and Surgeons, New York, NY

Johns Hopkins University School of Medicine, Baltimore, MD

New York University School of Medicine, New York, NY

Texas Tech University School of Medicine, Lubbock, TX

University of Missouri-Kansas City School of Medicine, Kansas City, MO

University of North Dakota School of Medicine, Grand Forks, ND

University of Texas Medical Branch at Galveston, Galveston, TX (UTSMDAC)

University of Texas Medical School at Houston, Houston, TX (UTSMDAC)

University of Texas Medical School at San Antonio, San Antonio, TX (UTSMDAC)

University of Texas Southwestern Medical School, Dallas, TX (UTSMDAC)

Yale University School of Medicine, New Haven, CT

If you're planning to apply to both AMCAS participating and non-participating medical schools, be sure to send away to the non-participating schools for application forms in plenty of time so that you can work comfortably on both the AMCAS materials and the non-AMCAS school's application forms. You'll be surprised at the amount of information necessary for these forms, and it would be wise not to wait until the last minute to begin.

I would strongly suggest that you obtain all the application materials in April or May at the latest and start looking them over right away. The earliest date your AMCAS application will be accepted is June 1. If you begin well before then, you'll have sufficient time to send for transcripts, send your application materials to AMCAS and non-AMCAS schools, and still be safe should AMCAS send back your application for revision if needed. Be sure to make note of each school's application deadlines, since a medical school won't accept individual applications afterward.

Number of Applications

The number of applications you send depends on several things. Firstly, the more medical schools you apply to, the better your odds become, up to a point. If all your credentials are poor, it doesn't matter how many schools you apply to; you probably won't be accepted to any. But if only one or two factors among your qualifications are below par, then there will probably be a few medical schools that will see you as a good candidate for their programs. Secondly, the cost of applying to many schools may prevent you from applying to as many as you would like. AMCAS charges an initial fee for the first school, with a decreasing fee scale for each additional school designated. A fee waiver form is provided to you as part of the packet you receive from AMCAS.

When applying to medical schools, be realistic in your self-evaluation, but never feel that you shouldn't apply to a particular school just because your credentials are not outstanding. Remember my student with the 2.5 GPA. We worked on her other qualifications for two years until she got in.

The next several chapters focus on the many different criteria medical schools use to evaluate candidates. What one medical school sees as important, another might not. Overall, however, the combination of grades and MCAT scores are the two most important factors. The following student ratings may help you in your selection decisions, but they shouldn't be used as a standard for every medical school.

Student Rating	GPA	MCAT Scores
Excellent	3.6 - 4.0	12 - 15
Very Good	3.4 - 3.5	10 - 11
Good	3.2 - 3.3	8 - 9
Average	3.0 - 3.1	6 - 7
Poor	2.0 - 2.9	1 - 5

Besides the two categories above, an excellent candidate would also have an outstanding record of extracurricular activities and very good letters of recommendation. These factors alone may put you into a higher category than you would otherwise be in with grades or MCAT scores alone. Again, don't hesitate to apply to any medical school you wish but, at the same time, keep in mind your realistic chances of success at some of the more prestigious schools.

Usually, the average number of medical schools an individual will apply to is 9. I knew one student who applied to 21 schools and didn't get accepted to any, and I also knew a student who'd applied to 4 schools and got accepted to all of them. Your chances depend on your credentials, your qualifications, your intangible factors, and the manner in which you present yourself on the interview. And because the average number of applications per student is 9, admission statistics and acceptance rates can be very deceptive. For example, at one medical school, 125 students were enrolled as freshman even though almost 300 acceptances were offered. At another "national" medical school, 200 students were enrolled as freshman but almost 400 were accepted. Those other accepted students chose to enter other medical schools or delayed their plans until the next year.

So, when you look at the percent of student enrollments at medical schools, keep in mind that any school has to accept at least twice as many students in order to fill their allotted class space. This means that instead of having a 1 in 5 or 1 in 10 chance of getting accepted to medical school, as some students think, any good student has a 1 in 2 chance of getting accepted if he or she plans wisely and chooses medical schools that are "good bets for success." Less prestigious schools, competing for students against better known schools, often have to accept as many as 60 percent of the applicants in order to fill their freshman quotas. Chances for admission, therefore, become much better if you plan your applications properly and if you're wise enough to apply to a selectively wide range of medical schools.

Reapplying to Medical School

According to several admissions committee members I'd spoken to, it's always a good idea to reapply to medical school several times if you're not accepted the first time. Many of the students I've helped over the years were accepted on the second or third try. One committee member even suggested reapplying 4 years in a row. There are several reasons for this:

1. Schools change deans of admission who have their own set of criteria for determining borderline cases. Your particular qualifications and/or credentials may be looked at in an entirely new light and can mean a big difference in terms of admissions policies for that year

2. Sometimes, a student's application may not be examined as thoroughly as it should be in any one particular year. One case I was told about involved a delay in the application screening process. When it was time to look at the mound of applications, the committee had to judge quickly and probably eliminated some students who might have gotten more consideration otherwise.

3. There's an entirely new pool of applicants each year with different backgrounds, credentials, and qualifications. Placing yourself with a new applicant pool can certainly affect your standing, sometimes in a negative way, but often in a better way, especially if you work on improving yourself during that year.

Being rejected by medical schools doesn't have to be the end of the road. From personal experience, I've known students who'd tried time and again before finally getting accepted because they persevered and especially because they worked on building stronger credentials. Medical schools can only look favorably on someone so determined to become a physician that he or she will keep improving in order to be accepted. Often, an extra year of preparation in one or two areas is all that's needed to make a difference between acceptance and rejection. So, rather than rush off to a foreign medical school or give up altogether, try reapplying a few times. If you're really serious about being in medicine, your desire will show through and your chances for acceptance will improve markedly.

Women Applicants

Over the years, the number of women applying to and being accepted to medical schools has grown tremendously. If the current trend continues, women applicants may even outnumber men by the next decade. The following is a sample of admissions statistics for women applicants over the last 50 years.

Year	Total Women Applicants	Number of Women Accepted
1950	1,390	385
1960	1,026	600
1970	2,289	1,297
1980	10,644	4,970
1985	12,476	5,705
1991	13,700	5,943
1993	17,957	7,288
1995	19,779	7,437
1997	18,273	7,485

In the past, attracting women was difficult because most women did not take the science and math required for admissions. Today, however, there are often as many women in math and science classes as there are men. Also, admissions committees in the past were set on "science" types whereas today non-science majors, as long as they complete the required courses for admission, are equally as qualified. Moreover, women have proven themselves to make excellent medical students and doctors, shattering the long-held belief that a medical career is too rigorous. So, regardless of what you might think your changes for admission to medical school are, don't let anything stop you from applying, if medicine is really what you want to do.

Age and the Applicant

Age is not an easy factor to discuss because different schools have different criteria regarding age limits. Legally, a medical school cannot discriminate based on age, but a medical school faculty member told me that if an admissions committee wants to keep you out they can do so very easily and make it look as if age had nothing to do with it. The good news is that, while it was customary in the past to accept mostly young students right out of college, today the average age of medical students is at least 25, with many incoming freshman in their 30s.

I've heard from several sources that the "unofficial" age limit for most schools is 35. This is based on the assumption that a person that age, if he or she practices until the age of 65, will still be in the medical profession for at least 20 years following graduation. Training a physician takes a lot of time and money and, naturally, medical schools would like their graduates to contribute many years of medical practice.

One premedical advisor, however, had told me that more medical schools are looking at the older applicant in a new light and with more flexibility than they ever have in the past. And because society is beginning to downplay age as a social issue - even accepting the fact that older individuals often make better students and more conscientious workers - medical schools are adjusting their thinking to reflect the views of society in general. In fact, the State University of New York at Buffalo had accepted a 55-year old woman, the oldest applicant ever to gain admission by that medical school.

Incoming freshman have more diverse backgrounds and work experience than ever before and, consequently, are older than they have been in the past. These applicants are viewed as more mature, stable, and experienced, qualities considered valuable during medical training. Another advisor also told me that this is true, but that the older applicant needs to be prepared to defend his or her decision to enter medicine much more so than younger applicants. Before going on the interview, older applicants should review all the positive aspects of their age and use that to their advantage. If they don't, the interviewers will certainly use age against them in their final evaluations.

The trend for acceptance of older applicants looks fairly good. While only 12 percent of applicants age 38 and older were accepted in 1978, almost 25 percent were accepted in 1986. In 1997-98 that number was closer to 30 percent. I believe the trend will continue as society becomes more aware of older individuals as members of society who have a great deal to offer as a result of experience, maturity, and incentive to strive for excellence.

Age can also be used to your advantage if you've participated in other than academic activities. Extracurricular activities such as work, family, church, and community organizations all show maturity, stability, responsibility, interest, concern, and involvement. In short, you'll be demonstrating a proven track record of fitness for medical school - something that a young individual may not have. So, don't think that age will hinder your chances for admission. With a little planning, thought, and foresight, you can turn your age into a positive quality that will make an admissions committee choose you, not in spite of your age, but because of it.

Letters of Evaluation

Depending on the medical school, you may be asked to supply three or more letters of recommendation from individuals who know you well or from the premedical advisory committee at your undergraduate institution. More and more medical schools are beginning to require a composite letter from a premedical evaluation committee (if there is one at your college or university) rather than individual letters. If your college has such a committee, but the medical school you're applying to will accept letters from either individuals or from a committee, definitely choose the committee. A medical school, naturally, would prefer a letter from an evaluations committee, and it would not look favorable on your part to opt for individual letters in that case. When discussing the letter with committee members, don't hesitate to ask them if there's any information they need from you in order to help them draft it.

Letters are valuable to admissions committees because they can offer the committee members an insight into your character and personality that they may not otherwise detect from your application or autobiographical sketch. For this reason, make every effort to become available and familiar to your advisory committee members without becoming a nuisance. I've seen students try so hard to get noticed by premedical faculty that they actually present a negative image. Don't be obnoxious. The best way to get to know faculty members is to pay them an occasional visit at an appropriate time (designated office hours) in order to discuss your plans and ask their advice. If a medical school or your premedical advisory committee requires letters from individuals, there are a few suggestions you should follow in order to make the best impression possible.

1. Make sure that you know the person well before asking for a letter of recommendation. A friend of mine was rejected by a genetic counseling firm even though she was well qualified simply because of a bad letter of recommendation. Apparently, the person writing the letter commented that she seemed immature and disagreeable. She learned the hard way that asking for a letter doesn't necessarily flatter someone into writing nice things about you. Be careful. More importantly, be selective.

2. Make sure that the individual writing the letter knows your character, personality, and motivation and would be willing to tell the admissions committee about the qualities you have which would make you a good physician. It's a waste to have someone who doesn't know you write a letter. When a student I've seen only once or twice asks me for letters of recommendation, I'll either refuse to do it or I'll write a general letter in which I actually say that I don't know this person all that well. Not a good reflection on you, as far as admissions committees go.

3. Don't be afraid to explain to the person writing the letter what medical schools are looking for in terms of qualifications, character, etc. Most individuals, especially if they're non-science types, are not familiar with medical school admissions criteria. Be honest and specify the kinds of things that an effective medical school letter should contain. Here are some particularly important characteristics to include:

   Personal Attributes: Discuss how the applicant interacts with other students and faculty members. Specify special characteristics which make the applicant suited for the study of medicine. Emphasize why the student has promise or potential for medicine. Use specific examples if possible rather than generalities.

   Academic Achievement: Without mentioning specific grades, emphasize why the student is capable of high academic achievement. Mention course difficulty, class standing, heavy course loads while also participating in extracurricular activities and/or work programs, student teaching, honors and awards, increasingly better GPA during upper level courses, etc.

   Overall Impressions and Evaluation: At the conclusion of the letter, a concise summary paragraph should contain a value judgment about the student's main strengths and why he or she would be an excellent candidate for medical school.

4. Don't ask teachers whose only contact with you has been a class or two to send letters. Admissions committee members can see for themselves whether or not you're a good student from your transcripts. They don't need to plod through a superficial letter by someone who hardly knows you outside of class. Sometimes, the winning quality an admissions committee is looking for is reflected by an individual who knows your personality well. If letters are to be sent by individuals, here are some good sources:

   Priest, rabbi, or minister who is personally familiar with your volunteer activities in church or in the community.

Supervisor or boss who can tell first hand about your motivation, work ethic, maturity, and dependability.

Close friend who is a respected professional such as a doctor, lawyer, banker, etc.

Most medical schools rely on letters of recommendation as one of the last criteria in making their selections. Sometimes, letters can be the deciding factor. It would be terrible if you failed to gain admission to medical school because you'd asked the wrong person to write a letter for you. Therefore, the two most important factors to consider as far as letters of recommendation go are: (1) know the person well, and (2) get acquainted with the premedical faculty and advisory committee at your college so that they know you personally.

Early Decision Program

The early decision program is a way for students to apply to one, and only one, school and receive an admission decision by October 1. The biggest advantage of this program is that you'll already know you've been accepted to a medical school and won't have to worry about applying to a lot of other schools. One other positive factor is that you'll save time and money by already having been accepted to the medical school of your choice.

Because the early decision program is a binding agreement between the applicant and the medical school, a student who decides not to accept an offer cannot accept any other offer from any other medical school. Therefore, you need to be sure that the medical school you choose is absolutely the right one for you.

The disadvantage of participating in the early decision program is that, if you're not accepted, you'll have to submit all your application materials to all other medical schools close to their application deadlines. This mad rush to get your applications in before the deadline is one of the worst things you can do. Since most of the early decision participating schools admit a very small percentage of their class through this program, I would recommend that you not apply for early decision unless you have all the following qualifications:

1. An overall GPA of 3.5 with a science GPA of at least 3.5

2. MCAT scores of at least 9 or 10 on each subsection of the exam

3. An outstanding record of extracurricular activities

4. Excellent letters of evaluation

5. Absolute certainty of the medical school you wish to attend

WICHE and WAMI Programs

These two programs enable students to enroll in out-of-state medical schools or other professional programs usually not available in their home states. WICHE is the Western Interstate Commission for Higher Education. Students from Alaska, Arizona, Idaho, Montana, Nevada, New Mexico, North Dakota, Utah and Wyoming can attend programs at reduced levels of tuition. The home state pays a support fee to the admitting school to help cover the cost of education.

Besides medicine, WICHE supports students interested in related health care fields such as dentistry, nursing, occupational therapy, optometry, osteopathic medicine, pharmacy, physical therapy, physician assistant, podiatry, public health, and veterinary medicine. To be eligible, a student must be a legal resident of one of the states participating. For more information write to:

Professional Student Exchange Program
Western Interstate Commission for Higher Education
P.O. Box 9752
1540 30th Street, RL-2
Boulder, CO 80301-9752

The WAMI program is designed to meet the educational needs of students from Washington, Alaska, Montana, Idaho, and Wyoming. In this program, students from these states are admitted to the University of Washington School of Medicine but take the first year of medical school at participating universities in their home states. These would be Washington State, University of Alaska, Montana State, University of Idaho, and the University of Wyoming. The curriculum at each site is compatible with the University of Washington medical school's curriculum. Admissions are handled completely by the University of Washington. For more information write to:

Director, WAMI Program
University of Washington School of Medicine
Seattle, WA 98195
(206) 543-7212

The Selection Factors

What are the main factors that admissions committees consider? We can group them into two main categories: (1) Objective data and (2) Subjective data. The objective data are academic performance measured either by GPA or an examination of individual transcripts to see the degree of difficulty of the course. The level of difficulty is compared with the amount of preparation the student had taken before taking the course. So, if you received a C in physics before taking any advanced math classes, that would explain your not getting a higher grade. Also considered in the selection decision is whether your academic performance had improved, leveled off, or got worse. It's not a good sign to see grades dropping.

The other objective data are the tests - MCAT, GRE, etc. These are convenient tools when a medical school is faced with literally thousands of applications. Unfortunately, schools with very large applicant pools will occasionally miss somebody who might otherwise be acceptable for medical school simply because of other qualifications.

The subjective data fall into several categories. Non-academic activities such as summer jobs and extracurricular involvement are very important and are discussed in more detail in the next chapter. All extra activities are balanced against academic performance. A person who has done nothing but study and get all A's might not be as strong a candidate as the person who had to work twenty hours or more a week to support himself in school, or had spent a good deal of time in community service, and has a B average instead of an A. Admissions committees also look at special talents and achievements that enable a student to be set apart from the large pool of applicants. Also important are letters of recommendation and how well a student presents him or herself on the interview.

One other subjective factor students seem to overlook is the interest that admissions committees might have in non-traditional fields. Most medical schools are concerned with the new disciplines that are becoming part of medicine. The social sciences and economics, for example, are becoming increasingly necessary in the health care delivery system. Systems analysts are also going to be important in medicine, as are biomedical engineers, bioethicists, and genetic counselors.

Many interests and disciplines have come along during the past decade that continue to add to and contribute to the practice of medicine. And as society becomes increasingly complex, the whole pattern of medical education and health care delivery will also continue to change. Medical schools can no longer admit only the stereotyped premed biology or chemistry major. What this means is that you now have an opportunity to make an impression on admissions committee members if your interests lie in a valuable and needed area of health care.

What Schools Are Best Bets For Successful Admission?

By far, your best chance of being accepted are with a medical school in your own state of residence. On average, state medical schools accept about 90 percent state residents and, therefore, will accept only a few, "very well qualified" non-resident applicants.

Even some of the privately-owned medical schools that receive financial assistance from the state they're located in are expected to accept a good percentage of state residents.

What it comes down to is that medical schools usually have two unofficial applicant pools: an in-state applicant pool and an out-of-state applicant pool. Because of higher entrance criteria, out-of-state applicants generally have higher GPAs and MCAT scores and, therefore, the in-state applicants would not do as well if they were compared with the usually more competitive out-of-state applicant pool. This doesn't mean that you shouldn't apply to any medical school you'd like, but you should realize that the odds are much more in your favor with schools in your own state of residence.

If you're well qualified (above average grades, high MCAT scores, excellent letters of evaluation, and a good record of extracurricular activities), then you may very well be a good candidate for one of the "national" schools such as Harvard, Duke, Johns Hopkins, etc. If your credentials are not superior, however, then your best bet is to look at schools in your own state and also at some of the less prestigious schools around the country which don't receive as many applications but which are trying to attract good quality students.

Remember, the larger the applicant pool, the less your chances become unless you're an outstanding candidate. Some of the better known medical schools receive as many as 5,000 applications a year and can certainly be more selective than a school receiving only 800. The former will almost always draw the line at grades and MCAT scores in order to cut the field down. So, if your grades and MCAT scores are not superior, your chances of getting very far into the selection process are slim.

If your primary goal is to become a doctor, but your qualifications are not the best, don't be so concerned about which medical school you'll be going to. Instead, concentrate your efforts on getting into a medical school period. Obtain a copy of the *Medical School Admission Requirements* and literature from individual medical schools. Examine your choices realistically according to your qualifications and the medical school's selection criteria. Talk to your premedical advisor about your chances of getting into a particular medical school and save yourself a lot of time and effort by choosing schools carefully and sensibly.

There are probably many good students who are not physicians today because they were either too narrow-minded about which school they wanted to attend or they didn't see their realistic chances of being accepted to certain medical schools. Let's face it; the student who seriously considers a career in medicine shouldn't be too concerned about the school's name on the diploma. How many times have you asked your doctor the name of the medical school he or she attended? Not many, I'm sure. When you begin practicing medicine, the name of the medical school you graduated from will very insignificant indeed.

In summary, then, when it comes down to which medical schools to apply to, we can list three basic strategies that are effective in boosting your overall probability for acceptance:

1. Unless you're in the top 10-20 percent of all students nationwide, you should always give first consideration to state-of-residence medical schools. Oddly enough, students still apply to medical schools that accept zero non-residents! Even someone in the top 1 percent isn't getting into those schools. Examine the ratios of resident to non-resident acceptance rates at medical schools and apply accordingly.

2. Be realistic when it comes to applying to nationally prestigious medical schools. I suspect that most students would like to attend Harvard, Yale, or Johns Hopkins. Realistically, very few have the credentials to even get through the initial screening process. Look carefully at your GPA, MCAT scores, background, and the competitiveness of your undergraduate institution. All things being equal, your undergraduate school is a key factor in how medical schools view the rest of your qualifications. The more competitive the undergraduate program, the better your chances become.

3. Always consider the stated mission of the medical school and how that mission fits in with your application profile. For example, a medical school's principle mission may be to train general practitioners for the state and would like applicants who have experience in the health care field. Even though you may have a good GPA and are a state resident, you may not "fit" the mission of the school or be suited to their program because you lack certain background qualifications. Before

applying to any school, review that school's brochure or catalogue and make sure your profile matches the aims and goals of that school. This can save you a lot of time and energy.

Applying For Residence Status

If you're serious enough about getting into medical school but just don't have the qualifications to compete against the better students, one alternative is to become a resident of a state with many medical schools. This would help your chances, since the vast majority of applicants come from the state in which the medical is located. How would a medical school react if you moved to a state in order to get into their program? In most cases, it would react favorably. Here are some reasons for applying for state residency:

1. You would join a state applicant pool that, in general, is probably not as academically well qualified as you would be. Normally, the out-of-state applicant pools have higher GPAs and MCAT scores than in-state applicant pools.

2. You would be increasing your chances of acceptance from 1 in 100 to 1 in 3 in some cases.

3. You would have employment for one year as a good life experience to include on your application

4. The medical school will see you as someone who is serious enough about medical school to be willing to relocate in order to gain admission.

To become a legal resident, you have to show that you came to that particular state with the true intention of becoming a legal resident. Residency requirements vary from state to state, but you would probably be assured legal resident status if you do the following:

- Get a job in that state
- File income tax as a state resident
- Get a state driver's license and registration
- Register to vote
- Open a savings and checking account
- Purchase property
- Establish credit within the state by opening charge accounts

Some Medical School Acceptance Records

In order to help you get an idea of which medical schools over the years have had the best acceptance records for non-residents, women, and minority students, I've included the following tables. Use these only as a guide in helping you make school selections, since admissions criteria change from year to year and from committee to committee. The latest edition of the AAMC's *Medical School Admission Requirements* will have the very latest statistics. However, never feel that you shouldn't apply to a particular school based only on statistics. Apply to any medical school you would like, but also apply to those schools that will give you a little extra insurance in terms of success rate. Unless specified, the following tables list schools in alphabetical order.

Medical Schools With Incoming Classes of 50 Percent or More Non-Residents

Albany Medical College
Albert Einstein College of Medicine
Boston University School of Medicine

Brown University School of Medicine

Columbia University College of Physicians and Surgeons

Cornell University Medical College

Creighton University School of Medicine

Dartmouth Medical School

Duke University School of Medicine

Finch University of Health Sciences / Chicago Medical School

George Washington University School of Medicine

Georgetown University School of Medicine

MCP/Hahnemann School of Medicine

Harvard Medical School

Howard University College of Medicine

Jefferson Medical College

Johns Hopkins University School of Medicine

Mayo Medical School

Meharry Medical College School of Medicine

Mount Sinai School of Medicine

New York Medical College

New York University School of Medicine

Northwestern University School of Medicine

Saint Louis University School of Medicine

Tufts University School of Medicine

Tulane University School of Medicine

University of Chicago Pritzker School of Medicine

University of Pennsylvania School of Medicine

University of Vermont College of Medicine

University of Washington School of Medicine

Vanderbilt University School of Medicine

Yale University School of Medicine

Medical Schools With Incoming Classes of 25 to 50 Percent Non-Residents

Baylor College of Medicine

Case Western Reserve University School of Medicine

Cornell University School of Medicine

Eastern Virginia Medical School

Emory University School of Medicine

Loma Linda University School of Medicine

Loyola University of Chicago Stritch School of Medicine

Medical College of Wisconsin

Morehouse School of Medicine

Oregon Health Sciences University School of Medicine

Pennsylvania State University College of Medicine

Stanford University School of Medicine

Temple University School of Medicine

University of Michigan School of Medicine

University of Missouri - Kansas City

University of North Dakota School of Medicine

University of Pittsburgh School of Medicine

University of Virginia School of Medicine

Virginia Commonwealth University School of Medicine

Wake Forest University School of Medicine

Thirty Medical Schools With the Highest Percentage of Incoming Women

Albert Einstein College of Medicine

Brown University School of Medicine

Columbia University College of Physicians and Surgeons

Cornell University Medical College

Howard University College of Medicine

Johns Hopkins University School of Medicine

Loyola University of Chicago Stritch School of Medicine

Meharry Medical College School of Medicine

Michigan State University College of Human Medicine

Morehouse School of Medicine

Mount Sinai School of Medicine

New York Medical College

Stanford University School of Medicine

SUNY - Stony Brook School of Medicine

Texas A&M University School of Medicine

Tulane University School of Medicine

University of California - San Francisco, School of Medicine

University of Buffalo School of Medicine and Biomedical Sciences

University of Connecticut School of Medicine

University of Florida School of Medicine

University of Hawaii School of Medicine

University of Louisville School of Medicine

University of Massachusetts Medical School

University of Miami School of Medicine

University of North Carolina at Chapel Hill School of Medicine

University of North Dakota School of Medicine

University of Vermont College of Medicine

University of Washington School of Medicine

Wake Forest University School of Medicine

Wright State University School of Medicine

Twenty-five Medical Schools With the Greatest Percentage of Minority Students

Brown University School of Medicine

Cornell University Medical College

Hahnemman School of Medicine

Harvard Medical School

Howard University College of Medicine

Meharry Medical College School of Medicine

Michigan State University College of Human Medicine

Morehouse School of Medicine

Stanford University School of Medicine

University at Buffalo School of Medicine and Biomedical Sciences

Temple University School of Medicine

University of California - Davis, School of Medicine

University of California - Irvine, School of Medicine

University of California - Los Angeles, School of Medicine

University of California - San Diego, School of Medicine

University of California - San Francisco, School of Medicine

University of Illinois College of Medicine

University of Medicine and Dentistry of New Jersey - New Jersey Medical School

University of Michigan Medical School

University of New Mexico School of Medicine

University of North Carolina at Chapel Hill School of Medicine

University of Texas Medical School at Galveston

University of Texas Medical School at San Antonio

Yale University School of Medicine

Medical Schools With the Highest Number of Applicants (5,000 or more; * = 7,500)

Albany Medical College *

Albert Einstein College of Medicine *

Boston University School of Medicine *

Case Western Reserve University School of Medicine

Cornell University Medical College

Creighton University School of Medicine

Dartmouth Medical College

Duke University School of Medicine

Emory University School of Medicine *

Finch University of Health Sciences/Chicago Medical School *

George Washington University School of Medicine and Health Sciences *

Georgtown University School of Medicine *

Howard University College of Medicine

Jefferson Medical College *

Loyola University of Chicago Stritch School of Medicine *

MCP/Hahnemann School of Medicine *

Medical College of Wisconsin

Mount Sinai School of Medicine *

New York Medical College *

Northwestern University School of Medicine *

Pennsylvania State University School of Medicine

Rush Medical College

St. Louis University School of Medicine

Stanford University School of Medicine

Temple University School of Medicine *

Tulane University School of Medicine *

Tufts University School of Medicine *

University of California - Los Angeles, School of Medicine

University of California - San Francisco, School of Medicine

University of Chicago Pritzker School of Medicine *

University of Michigan Medical School

University of Pennsylvania School of Medicine *

University of Pittsburgh School of Medicine

University of Southern California School of Medicine

University of Vermont College of Medicine

University of Washington (St. Louis) School of Medicine

Vanderbilt University School of Medicine

Wake Forest University School of Medicine

Summary of Schedule for the Application Process

1. See your premedical advisor about the premedical program and make sure you understand the requirements completely.

2. Take required courses for medical school admissions and especially those that will prepare you for the MCAT.

3. Register for and take the MCAT one year before you plan on entering medical school

4. Take the MCAT in the spring (preferably) or the fall.

5. Obtain application materials from both AMCAS and from non-AMCAS schools at least one month before the earliest application date.

6. Have all transcripts sent to AMCAS and to non-AMCAS schools you apply to.

7. Begin filling out application materials in plenty of time before the earliest deadline.

8. Send application materials to AMCAS (after June 1) and to non-AMCAS medical schools as soon after their earliest filing dates as possible.

9. Wait for medical schools to reply and let you know that additional supplementary forms and letters are required.

10. Send supplementary application forms (provided by the medical schools) and have letters sent directly to the medical school.

11. Wait to be called for an interview, then go on the interview well prepared and calm.

12. Wait for an acceptance or rejection letter.

13. Notify the medical school of your decision to accept their offer for admission and send the appropriate deposit which will hod your place in class. Your acceptance to attend one school doesn't mean you can't accept any other offers. If a better school accepts you, you can get your previous deposit back, providing you notify the school in the allotted time period.

Sample of an Autobiographical Sketch from a Successful Applicant

Born in Jefferson, North Carolina, I was raised with two younger sisters and a younger brother. My grandfather owns a farm, and my father, being an only son, took over the family farm after my grandfather suffered a stroke nearly five years ago. Even before that incident, though, I had always been involved in farm work, mostly tending cattle and growing tobacco. For the past three years, I've also been in charge of taking care of more than 4,000 Christmas trees, which take up much of my time while I'm at home. I think of my trees more as a hobby than a chore, since I really enjoy the opportunity of being out by myself on a piece of the farm I consider my very own.

Because of my closeness with my family, and my responsibilities to the farm, I try to go home nearly every weekend. Until recently, I have been the only pianist at my church and am depended upon to be there every Sunday. My two sisters and my brother, who I try to see as much as possible, also give me an added reason for visiting often. My grandfather, now in a wheelchair because of his stroke, still has his car and only gets to ride in it when I'm there to drive him.

In making my decision to apply to medical school, I have continually debated with myself about what is required of a doctor and whether or not this is a career for me. I have always thought of a doctor as both a scientist and a social worker, two professions I've always had a desire to enter. Socially, I have always been active in my community and my church. Being the leader of my youth group, I've worked closely with my pastor in planning county-wide youth events and visiting the sick and needy, especially during Christmas.

I have worked many different jobs, always learning to deal with a different group of people. Working as a pharmacy drug clerk in the lower working class section of Winston-Salem has given me confidence that I have the ability to deal with sick and often frightened people. My volunteer work at North Carolina Baptist Hospital has also given me an insight into what caring for the sick and dying is all about. When dealing with and caring for my grandfather, I had to show both strength and compassion because the attitude I had toward him would have determined how he looked and how he felt about his handicap. If there is one personal quality that I would extend to my work as a doctor, it would be my willingness to touch the lives of my patients in a sincere and human way. I think that it's essential for a doctor to deal with people on a one-to-one basis, and my work has given me the opportunity to learn just that.

Love of science has also affected my decision to apply to medical school. After being a volunteer in surgery research at Wake Forest University School of Medicine, I decided to do undergraduate research in chemistry. I soon found out that success, and sometimes failure, are part of a learning process, and that we all need to accept our failures in order to become more successful and better human beings.

In thinking about a medical career, I've come to realize that there's an increasing need for doctor's who are willing to serve small town hospitals and rural communities. I also realize that the reward for serving these hospitals and communities is not so much financial as it is a personal satisfaction. Knowing this has not discouraged me from my principle career goal: to serve those communities and their people in the best way I possibly can, as a family physician in a rural community.

6

Extracurricular Activities

Because there are more well-qualified applicants than ever seeking entrance into U.S. medical schools, admissions committees need to go beyond grades and MCAT scores to distinguish between good and exceptional candidates. One of the ways they do this is by looking at extracurricular activities. Extracurricular activities can be anything outside your normal course of study such as employment, volunteer work, community service, sports, political involvement, etc.

Any kind of outside activity reveals to an admissions committee something about your character, your interest in people, and your sincere desire to be involved with others. In essence, what you do outside the classroom environment says a lot about you and will indicate to the medical school what kind of person you really are. Even if you're an introvert, force yourself to get involved, and never underestimate the importance outside activities will have on your success as a potential candidate.

Importance of Non-Academics

So far, I've discussed the academic side of premedical planning without going into the non-academic side, which can be equally as important if you're really serious about becoming a successful applicant. What kinds of extracurricular activities should you become involved with in order to enhance your chances for acceptance? And what do medical schools look for in particular when examining an applicant's non-academic credentials? Many students don't consider these two questions, which need to be addressed in order to make one's application as appealing as possible.

A friend of mine once told me that her brother was rejected by a state medical school because he didn't have enough extracurricular activities on his record. He was a typical bookworm, never becoming involved in anything but school work. So he spent the next year doing volunteer work, reapplied, and eventually got accepted the second time around. Don't make the mistake other students make; that scholastic excellence alone will assure you a place in medical school. Start thinking about getting involved in non-academic activities now. When admissions committees look at students with very high GPAs (3.8 - 4.0), they also look very closely at their outside interests. What they often find is that many of these students are overly competitive and don't get involved in anything other than studying.

After talking to many committee members, I strongly recommend that you devote more time to developing a wide scope of interests rather than worrying about getting a 3.95 GPA. Until they begin to get rejection letters, premedical students can't seem to get it into their heads that the difference between a 3.5 and a 4.0 GPA is often insignificant as far as an admissions committee is concerned. What *is* important is what you've done while maintaining a 3.5 GPA. The following are some areas of involvement that have been successful for many of the students I've spoke to and which I feel would be positive factors during the selection process.

Athletics

It's difficult to maintain good grades while participating in school athletics. This is one reasons why you should emphasize this aspect of your college life, especially if you've been involved in varsity sports. Two individuals I knew who were on the wrestling team easily gained admission to medical school mainly because their grades were high and the medical schools they'd applied to knew how difficult a wrestling schedule is.

Other sports activities such as football, baseball, swimming, and track, which require students to be away from school and classes at times, are also looked at as good character and team player builders. Admissions committees assume that, if these students maintain high grades despite their rigorous travel times and practices, they would certainly be able to handle the medical school schedule. Naturally, other factors are considered before athletics, but athletics can be a very positive item on your list of activities.

Academic Clubs and Organizations

Any club or organization you may belong to will look make your application look better than not belonging to any organization at all. Admissions committees look at your participation as a sign of your involvement with other individuals. A physician is constantly involved with people, and this part of your premedical preparation is seen as a good training period for the interrelationships you'll be experiencing during your medical practice.

Debating Team

This activity always looks good on your application because a good physician must also be an effective communicator. If you're a straight A student but you can't communicate your ideas in a clear manner, you might as well forget medical school. Many upper division classes in medical school require oral reports and presentations before classmates and other faculty members. Even some of the examinations are given orally. Being on the debating team will demonstrate confidence, poise, and the ability to relate ideas in a coherent and convincing manner. What better quality for a doctor to have than the ability to explain a prognosis or diagnosis to a patient or to a team of medical professionals.

Many physicians are involved in teaching, both on a salaried and volunteer basis. At the medical school I was associated with, numerous seminars are given each day by physicians and students involved in clinical and scientific research. Being able to present the growing amount of scientific information to the general public, as well as to the medical sector, is an important part of today's health professional. Showing admissions committee members that you have this quality will surely improve your standing as a potential medical school candidate.

Science Clubs

Although being a science major is not a prerequisite for medical school, there's still one major conclusion many medical school faculty persistently acknowledge: that, in order to be a good doctor, you need to be a good scientist. Medicine is a discipline based on scientific information, observation, and sometimes experimentation, and because of that, an individual must be able to examine ideas and concepts critically and interpret results according to scientific principles. As a member of a scientific club, you would be demonstrating a desire to actively involve yourself in the field of science. If you participate in any projects or volunteer work, make sure you mention so in your application so that the admissions committee will be able to see your enthusiasm for scientific work.

Alpha Epsilon Delta

Many schools have chapters of AED, which is an honor society for preprofessional students. The activities associated with membership vary from chapter to chapter but, in general, the activities include:

- Volunteer work at local hospitals, the Red Cross, and other health-related organizations.
- Trips to medical schools to see their facilities and faculty members.
- Seminars and lectures by physicians, medical faculty, and other health professionals
- MCAT review sessions
- Meetings and outings with other students and premedical faculty members and advisors

Non-participation in AED is not something admissions committees frown upon but, by the same token, membership may signal your genuine interest in learning more about the medical profession. There's an annual membership fee, but the price is insignificant compared to the possible impact your involvement in AED could make on an admissions committee, as well as the premedical committee at your college or university. I feel that the greatest advantage of membership is the contact you'll make with individuals who will be writing letters.

Student Projects

Many faculty members are involved in research projects and welcome the opportunity to have some volunteer assistance. If you have an area of interest (genetics, biochemistry, physiology, etc.), talk to the faculty members in those departments, find out if they're currently doing any research projects, and whether or not they're willing to take on a volunteer student. Make sure you tell them that you're offering your services for free, since they probably won't have money budgeted for you and won't be interested.

Volunteer Work

This area of your credentials is especially important, since it shows that you're willing to give of yourself and are demonstrating your willingness to meet the needs of others. Volunteer work can be done in school and/or the community and especially looks good when it involves interaction with people. As a doctor, after all, you'll have to deal with people constantly. Here are some examples of volunteer activities you may want to get involved in and which have been shown to impress medical school admission committee members:

School projects	Community outreach programs
Tutoring	Boy / Girl Scouts
Student government	Big Brother / Sister Program
Student newspaper	CPR / First Aid Instructor
Science clubs	Church activities
Orchestra / Band	Community action groups
Athletics	Hospital work

A friend of mine related a story to me about his interview at a midwestern medical school a few years back. The person interviewing him asked if he had any inclination for a certain area or specialty of medicine. My friend immediately replied that he wanted to go into pediatrics because he loved children and enjoyed working with juveniles. The interviewer looked at my friend's records, which showed that he'd been involved in the Big Brother's Program for a number of years, and told him that he would make a fine pediatrician. There was no doubt that my friend's involvement in that program made an impression on the interviewer and was an important factor in his being accepted to 3 out of 4 medical schools he'd applied to.

Employment

Regardless of the type of job you've had or have now, whether it's full or part-time, seasonal or annual, it's important to include this part of your history on your application. Medical schools expect their students to work hard – harder than they've ever worked before. Someone who can maintain a good GPA while working full or part-time will make a good candidate for medical school. It really doesn't matter what kind of work you've done (although health-related work will look great) as long as you've been a conscientious worker and have kept up your grades.

Often, an admissions committee will examine grades keeping your employment in mind. If you've worked your way through school, for example, your grades may not be a true reflection of your potential. Always include any employment experience you've had during high school or college since this shows that you've at least learned reliance, gained life experience, and possess motivation.

Intangible Selection Factors

Probably the four most important intangible factors medical schools look for when screening applicants are maturity, leadership, motivation, and sincerity. All these characteristics can be demonstrated by the activities you involve yourself with or the jobs you've held while in school and are expected in someone who will have an M.D. degree. Answer the following questions associated with each factor and see how much you need to improve your intangible qualities. If you possess many of these qualities, then you're exactly the king of person medical schools hope to attract.

Maturity

Have I demonstrated my maturity by holding a full or part-time job while attending school?

Can I give specific examples of my ability to work with others and my ability to be dependable, conscientious, and responsible?

Did I accomplish anything of significance (in any field or activity) during my undergraduate years?

Have I ever shown that I'm able to cope with adverse life situations?

Have I ever had to perform under pressure or work closely with others in order to meet deadline, etc.?

If I'm married, am I still able to be a successful student and maintain a healthy married life?

Do I have to support a family?

Have I held any positions in school or in the community that require a mature, responsible individual?

Have I served in the armed forces?

Leadership

Have I belonged to organizations that served the needs of the community, my school, or my church?

Have I held any positions of leadership that required my supervision or decision-making?

Have I ever served in a supervisory capacity at a civilian job or in military service?

Have I ever been required to analyze problems and make decisions or judgements in order to solve those problems?

Have I ever held positions requiring use of communicative skills (presenting oral reports, writing papers, etc.)?

Have I been the leader of a group such as the Boy Scouts?

Have I been an instructor of some kind (CPR, first aid, sports, tutoring, etc.)?

Motivation

Have I had to overcome obstacles (physical, financial, emotional) in order to complete school?

Can I give examples of my ability to achieve an end result because of my self-confidence, stamina, and perseverance?

Have I taken night classes while working during the day?

Did I have to work nights after going to school during the day?

Did I attend summer school?

Have I worked on special research projects in my major field or outside my curriculum?

Have I done much laboratory volunteer work?

Can I, with self-assurance, describe how my interest in medicine developed and how my past life experience will make me a better physician?

Sincerity

Have I done volunteer work at a hospital, nursing home, the Red Cross, or any other health-related organization?

Do I belong to any premedical fraternities, clubs, or organizations?

Have I demonstrated in any way that I chosen a career in medicine in order to meet the needs of others and am willing to devote my life to helping the sick?

Naturally, many of these qualities can fall under more than one category. The main point is that you need to start thinking about the non-academic part of your education if you're going to be a truly good candidate for medical school. If you seriously make a commitment to be the kind of person that medical schools want, then you need to get involved right now. Don't wait until you junior year, because admission committee members have the experience to recognize a person who simply tries to pad their resume with extracurricular work at the last minute to impress them.

Besides, the pleasure you'll receive from contributing your time and efforts to the service of others will give you a taste of the rewards you'll receive when you finally begin practicing medicine. Hospital work will also give you a true indication of whether you would really like spending the better part of your life around sick people. Admissions committees will see this as attempt on your part to experience medicine first-hand before making a serious commitment to medical school.

Two points worth mentioning: (1) Regardless of your extracurricular record, never allow your grades to suffer too much and (2) be committed in your extracurricular work – don't just do it to get something on your application. Even though grades are often not the final deciding factor, be careful that your GPA does not slip below a 3.3 (3.5 if you're serious about applying to top schools). Once your GPA gets too low, no amount of outside activity will get you past that initial screening process in many schools.

As long as your grades and MCAT scores are good enough to make it through the first round (very important), your extracurricular activities should seal your acceptance. Also, make sure that you don't do what many unsuccessful applicants do – participate in an absurd number of activities that are meant only to fill up their application. Again, admissions committees are looking for dedicated individuals who contribute something to whatever they're involved in

Extracurricular Survey

The following is a survey I'd taken of incoming freshman medical students. I did it to find out from the students themselves what they thought helped them most in gaining admission to medical school. Following each question are the answers along with the number of students giving those answers. More than one answer was possible for each student.

Q. During college, what types of extracurricular activities did you participate in?

Hospital volunteer work	86
Athletics	82
Fraternities	72
Social committees	56
Employment (full or part-time)	46
Alpha Epsilon Delta	42
Student government	36
Service organizations	28

Science clubs	26
Honor societies	16
Student newspaper	8
Scuba club	2
Glee club	2
Theatrical club	1

Q. What quality or qualities do you feel contributed most to your being accepted to medical school?

Grade Point Average (GPA)	96
Motivation	72
Hospital experience	51
High MCAT scores	48
Good interview	40
Good recommendations	32
Volunteer work (general)	26
Sincerity	26
Maturity	22
Non-science major	3
Traveling experience	2

Q. What quality or personal attribute do you think will help you most during your first year as a medical student?

Motivation	78
Maturity	75
Ability to work hard	72
Intelligence	53
Past experiences	25
Other	20

Many of the surveyed medical students participated in or were involved in several extracurricular activities. The "common denominator" among these successful students seemed to be their non-academic credentials, and I would be inclined to say that a student with average grades (3.0 GPA) but an outstanding record of non-academic involvement has a better chance of getting into medical school than a student having high grades but nothing else.

The lesson here is that the non-academic side of your overall credentials is just as important for successful admission and should be taken seriously. Students who are medical schools today are the ones who learned early on what was expected of them both academically and non-academically and may not necessarily have been any more qualified than some rejected applicants. Don't throw away your future because someone else knew the inside strategy and gets accepted ahead of you. I've known quite a few students who theoretically should never have been accepted but who were simply because they knew how to take advantage of every opportunity available to them. So get the competitive edge by being involved in more than just academics. Become that special student every medical school is looking for.

7

Medical College Admissions Test

With a few exceptions, the majority of medical schools require that you take the MCAT as a prerequisite for admission. The exam is given twice a year, in April and in August throughout testing sites in the United States. Medical schools prefer that you take the MCAT during the spring of the year before you plan to enter. In this way, scores will get to the schools in plenty of time and you'll still be able to retake the exam in the fall without reapplying to medical school should you decide that your scores were not as good as you'd expected. Medical schools will, in fact, give acceptance priority to spring MCAT students because their admissions materials are already on file. For example, if you wish to start medical school in the fall 2000, you should take the MCAT in spring 1999 or, at the latest, the fall of 1999.

About the MCAT

Designed by the Association of American Medical Colleges (AAMC), the MCAT is an all-day, 6-hour exam consisting of four sections: (1) Verbal Reasoning, (2) Physical Sciences, (3) Writing Sample, and (4) Biological Sciences. Examinees arrive at the test site at 8 a.m. and begin the exam at 9 a.m. Typically, the exam ends about 4 p.m. The MCAT schedule is as follows:

SECTION	NUMBER OF QUESTIONS	ALLOTED TIME
Verbal Reasoning	65	85 minutes
Break		10 minutes
Physical Sciences	77	100 minutes
Lunch Break		60 minutes
Writing Sample	2	60 minutes
Break		10 minutes
Biological Sciences	77	100 minutes

The MCAT is not like any exam you've ever taken before. It's extremely challenging, consisting of various passages that test a student's ability to analyze data, interpret results, and understand information presented in tables, graphs, and charts. A separate score is awarded for each of the four sections, and the scores are then sent to you and the medical schools you designate on the application form 6-7 weeks following the test.

For the Verbal Reasoning, Physical Sciences, and Biological Sciences, the raw score (number of correct answers) is converted to a scale ranging from a low of 1 to a high of 15. The final score is a "curve" of how the entire group did on that particular test and it indicates how much above or below average your raw test score was. Typically, a score of 8 is the national average for each section, a score of 12 puts you in the top 2 percent nationally, a 15 corresponds to the 99th percentile. The writing sample is scored from a low of 1 to a high of 6 and is described below. The sections measure and evaluate several areas of performance:

Verbal Reasoning: This section consists of 9 passages of 500-600 words each and determines a student's ability to understand and evaluate information in arguments related to humanities, social sciences, and natural sciences. The questions measure comprehension, evaluation, applying knowledge, and incorporating new information.

Physical Sciences: This section, composed of 77 multiple choice questions, tests reasoning skills in physics and general chemistry. Most of the questions are based on problem sets of 5-10 questions per set. Some of the sets will have tables and/or graphs. The remaining questions are independent of any problem set. This part of the MCAT measures general science knowledge, research interpretation, and problem solving ability in physics and chemistry. A 60 minute lunch break follows.

Writing Sample: Taken right after lunch, the writing sample section consists of two 30-minute essays designed to assess writing skills. When grading essays, scorers look at your ability to develop a central theme, synthesize concepts, organize an answer, explain the statement, and present ideas in a clear and coherent manner. Essay topics are never controversial (no religion or politics), nor will they require prior knowledge of a particular subject. Scores of 1-6 are awarded, with 1 being lowest (totally failed to address the topic; obvious problems with organization, language, etc.) and 6 the highest (thorough treatment; focused, coherent, clear, superior vocabulary, grammar, and sentence structure). The raw scores are determined by two graders, then summed and converted to an alphabetical scale ranging from J (lowest) to T (highest)

Biological Sciences: This last section measures knowledge of the biological sciences and organic chemistry. Like the physical sciences section, the 62 questions are based on passages and 15 independent multiple choice questions.

How MCAT Scores Are Interpreted

Most admissions committees use MCAT scores together with GPA and other factors to determine a point total for an applicant. Different schools vary in how they interpret MCAT scores, some placing more emphasis on grades, others on science GPA and the science sections of the MCAT, still others on non-science or overall GPA and the verbal reasoning and writing sample. Most schools, however, place a great deal of weight on the MCAT, especially since the questions are designed, not so much to test one's ability to regurgitate learned information but to think and reason critically, which is vital to doing well in medical school classes.

The MCAT is also used to validate your GPA and compare it with applicants from hundreds of different undergraduate schools. If your GPA is high but your MCAT scores are low, for example, it may indicate that your grades were inflated or that your background is not as strong as it should be. Since the exam is written specifically at the biology, chemistry, and physics "introductory" level, all applicants should be equally prepared for it, whether they've taken advanced courses or not. In fact, it's better to learn the basics very, very well than to take a lot of advanced classes just for the sake of taking them.

The examination fee entitles the applicant to send test scores to as many as six non-AMCAS medical schools, as well as any AMCAS schools applied to. A fee waiver is granted for those with financial difficulties. The MCAT information booklet, which includes application materials, sample questions, and fee information is available from:

MCAT Program Office
P.O. Box 4056
Iowa City, IA 52243

As with everything else, MCAT scores are only one factor (albeit an important one) that admissions committees examine when selecting applicants. However, it may be very important if you're set on attending a private or an out-of-state medical school as a non-resident. In that case, your MCAT scores better be higher than average.

Like GPA, MCAT scores range widely within an incoming class because other criteria come into play which outweigh a low score on the MCAT. High scores, though, will certainly help your chances for admission if some other aspect of your academic record is inadequate. In order to ensure success, you should have as many positive factors in your file as possible. If all your credentials are good, then good MCAT scores will surely improve your chances even more.

Since the new MCAT was introduced in April, 1991, scores have remained relatively stable. Here are the statistics for "accepted" applicants from 1992 to 1997. The scores for the total applicant pool was, on average, 1 point lower.

Section	1992	1993	1994	1995	1996	1997
Verbal Reasoning	9.2	9.4	9.4	9.5	9.6	9.6
Physical Sciences	9.2	9.3	9.4	9.7	9.9	9.8
Writing Sample	3	4	4	4	4	4
Biological Sciences	9.3	9.5	9.6	9.8	10.0	10.1

Even though MCAT scores are important, when a survey of medical school admissions personnel was taken, it was found that the MCAT data was looked at much differently, depending on the applicant. For example, 40 percent of the respondents said they placed greater emphasis on test scores for students graduating from unfamiliar or less competitive undergraduate institutions, 30 percent felt that non-residents needed higher scores than residents, and 70 percent said they evaluated test scores for minority and/or disadvantaged students differently than they did for majority applicants. Some compared minority applicant scores to the national mean for minority applicants alone and said they would accept lower test scores as long as other evidence of academic success and potential were there. Others looked only at the last set of scores while a few looked at a combination of scores to get a better idea of a student's potential and/or progress. Regardless of how they examine MCAT results, most admissions committees look for reasons why scores might be low, such as low academic potential or insufficient preparation before the exam.

Retaking the MCAT

How do you know whether or not to retake the exam? And how many times? First of all, you should consult with your premedical advisor. He or she has had enough experience with accepted and rejected students to know how different schools react to certain MCAT scores. Normally, scores don't differ much unless there was a serious deficiency in one of the subjects included on the exam. Only you can judge whether or not additional preparation will help. Repeating the MCAT without showing much improvement is not going to be looked at favorably by admissions committee members and can work against you. So, before making a decision to retake the exam, you need to be serious. Your scores must improve or you must have demonstrated some other outstanding achievement that will enhance your overall application.

If you've taken the MCAT three or more times, you must apply for special permission to take the MCAT again. Your request needs to include evidence of your intent to apply to medical school such as a completed application, letter of rejection, or a letter from a medical school or premedical advisor. This must be done each time you wish to retake the exam.

One of the reasons students in their junior year do poorly on the spring MCAT and need to retake it is poor preparation. Once these students realize how rigorous the MCAT is, they prepare more diligently and usually do better. I always recommend to my students to prepare for at least 3 months, preferably six. If you or your advisor decide that your scores are not competitive enough, then use the first set of scores as a guide to pinpoint areas of weakness. For example, if you did well on everything except the physical sciences section, concentrate your efforts on improving those areas. Retake a class or sit in on some lectures. Spend your time wisely by studying those topics that gave you the most trouble. Here are some good reasons for retaking the MCAT:

1. Not having the introductory science classes necessary to understand the questions on the exam.

2. A wide discrepancy between MCAT scores and GPA.

3. An admissions committee member suggesting that scores are too low to be realistically competitive.

4. An illness at the time of the exam that effected your ability to concentrate properly.

How To Prepare For the MCAT

No matter what I tell students, there's always a misconception about how in-depth the science questions get. This cause a great deal of anxiety, especially for students who aren't science majors or who haven't taken many science courses other than the prerequisites. It's important to remember that it's not necessary to take advanced classes, although in some cases taking a few extra science courses seems to reinforce what has been learned already. This doesn't mean you shouldn't take advanced courses if you really want to; it simply means that if you prepared well in all your introductory biology, chemistry, and physics courses, and understood the material well, you should be at the same level of preparedness as anyone else.

Should you take a commercial MCAT preparation course? For some students, it's not necessary, and may even be a waste of money. For others it's money well spent. What many of these preparation programs do is help students organize and review basic introductory science materials, as well as teach them "how" to take the exam, since it's different than any other exam most students have ever taken. Kaplan, for example, offers a comprehensive study program, as does the Columbia Review and Betz. A good course will include actual questions from previous MCATs in order for you to get a feel for the types of passages and questions that will be asked.

Often, the difference in MCAT performance is the amount of time students spend preparing. They take the exam for granted, thinking that as long as they've done well in their classes they'll do well on the exam. Not so. Most students never see exams that require them to analyze data, interpret graphs and research results, or think critically. If anything, the MCAT is an indicator of your ability to use the thought process to solve problems. A good commercial preparation course will at least help you get used to seeing those types of questions. Regardless of whether you take a commercial course or not, here are three important things to do when preparing:

1. Be ready to "review" for the MCAT, not see the material for the first time. In other words, it's essential that you've taken the necessary coursework before you study. Learning new material while reviewing is difficult at best, especially if you're also taking other classes at the same time.

2. Be disciplined and organized. Without these, review sessions can be a waste of time and will result in poor MCAT scores. Set specific times aside, and stick to those times. Your mind and body will automatically gear up for study sessions if you're consistent.

3. Determine how well you've learned previous material before you attempt an independent review. If necessary, sitting in on some lectures or even retaking a class can be an advantage. Remember, the MCAT only includes basic materials. Concentrate on those.

Getting Ready for the Physical Sciences and Biology Sections

These sections are important because many admissions committee members feel, naturally so, that medicine requires one to be good at solving scientific problems. Here are some helpful hints and ideas that will help you in getting ready.

- Students who take chemistry and physics as soon before the MCAT as possible usually do better. Furthermore, review will be easier since the material will still be fresh in their minds.

- Plan on taking chemistry and physics early enough so that you have at least 3 months to review. Don't assume that you can take the MCAT while still taking those courses.

- Many schools with good premedical programs have a set of review tapes and notes in their testing centers which you can use or rent during your preparation. Utilize them.

- Obtain several different MCAT study manuals and work through them carefully. They're especially helpful in getting you accustomed to the format of the exam and in preparing you for the length of time the exam takes. It's important that you time yourself carefully and spend the entire day taking the exam, just as you would at the testing center.

- Use class notes as well as other sources such as introductory textbooks to help you review general concepts. Sometimes looking at several different texts will help you see the material in a new, and sometimes clearer, light.

- Obtain the latest MCAT study guide published by the AAMC in order to review the topics to be covered on the next exam.

- Keep a separate notebook and jot down any information you come across that you don't know and that will be part of the topic area covered on the MCAT. For example, some of the information you'll encounter in MCAT study manuals and other sources may not have been covered well in your classes by any of your teachers. Don't assume that college professors include all the material considered important by MCAT test preparers.

- Use index cards to write down critical formulas, important concepts, and important chemical structures. Use these as flash cards to imprint that information in your mind before the exam.

Key Science Terms

The following is a list of important biology, chemistry, and physics terms you should go through as you prepare for the MCAT. Don't be satisfied with knowing only the meanings of these terms. Make sure you understand the concepts as well as any theories that may be associated with them. For example, when you get to the term "aldehydes" under the chemistry section, you should not only know what an aldehyde is, you should also be able to solve problems dealing with reactions of aldehydes, nomenclature of aldehydes, and the conversion of aldehydes to primary and secondary alcohols. In short, spend your time studying and reviewing the key science terms in detail rather than going over any superficial meanings. Some terms are common to several fields such as biology *and* chemistry. Terms not found in the biology terms section may be found in the chemistry section.

Biological Science Terms

acclimatization	acetylcholine	acromegaly
acrosome	ACTH	actin
action potential	activation energy	active transport
adaptive radiation	Addison's disease	ADH
ADP	adenine	adrenal cortex
adrenal medulla	adrenaline	afferent
aldosterone	algae	allantois
allele	allopathic	alveolus
amnion	amylase	amphibian
anabolism	anaerobic	anaphase
androgen	anemia	angiosperm
angiotensin	annelid	anthozoa
antibody	anticodon	antigen
aorta	apocrine	apnea
aqueous humor	arachnid	archenteron
artery	arteriosclerosis	arthropod
ascomycetes	astigmatism	atrium

atrophy

autotrophic

bacillus

basidiomycetes

binary fission

blastodisc

blind spot

Bohr effect

Brunner's gland

calcitonin

CAM

catalysis

cell theory

centriole

cerebellum

chemotaxis

chief cells

cholesystokinin

chorion

chromosome

chymotrypsin

climax community

coelom

conjugation

cretinism

cytochrome

cytosine

diabetes

diploid

dominance

ectoderm

endoderm

epiboly

epistasis

estrus

extensor

follicle

gamete

genotype

glucagon

glucose

goblet cell

gonad

autonomic nervous system

AV node

bacteriophage

bile

biological clock

blastopore

blood clotting mechanism

Bowman's capsule

bryophyte

Calvin Cycle

cardiac output

catecholamines

cellulose

centrosome

cerebrospinal fluid

chemosynthesis

chloroplast

chordata

chromatid

chromosome map

cistron

codominance

commensalism

convergence

cristae

cytokinesis

dendrite

diastole

divergent evolution

dorsal lip

efferent

endoplasmic reticulum

epididymus

erythroblastosis

eucaryotic

fermentation

free martin

gastrin

glial cell

glucocorticoid

glycogenolysis

goiter

gonadotropin

autosomes

axon

Barr body

bilirubin

blastocoel

blastula

blood groups

bronchi

budding

calyx

catabolism

cell cycle

central nervous system

centromere

cerebrum

chiasmata

cholesterol

chorioallantoic membrane

chromatin

chyme

cleavage

codon

cones

corpus luteum

crossing over

cytoplasm

deuterosome

diffusion

DNA

EKG

endocrine

enzyme

epinephrine

erythropoiesis

exocrine

flexor

FSH

gastrula

glomerulus

gluconeogenesis

glycolysis

golgi

gram staining

guanine

hermaphrodite

heterothermic

homeothermic

hyaline

hypertension

hypothalamus

imprinting

insulin

isolecithal

jaundice

Klinefelter's syndrome

loop of Henle

lysosome

malleus

medulla

mesoderm

metaphase

mitochondria

murmur

natural selection

niche

nucleolus

organ of Corti

ovulation

parathyroid hormone

partial pressure

phagocytosis

phyla

placenta

platelet

polar bodies

procaryotic

protoplasm

purkinje fibers

radial symmetry

REM

resting potential

RNA

sarcolemma

schizomycetes

semicircular canals

spermatogenesis

haploid

hematocrit

heterozygous

homologous

hyaluronidase

hypertonic

hypotonic

infarction

ischemia

isometric

karyokinesis

Krebs cycle

Leydig cells

macula densa

marrow

meiosis

metabolism

midbrain

mitosis

mutualism

nephron

norepinephrine

nucleus

organizer

oxygen debt

parietal cells

pepsinogen

phenotype

pinocytosis

plasma

pleiotrophy

polygenic inheritance

prophase

pulmonary

pyrimidine

recessive

renin

rods

sarcomere

sclera

sex linkage

spindle fibers

stapes

Hardy-Weinberg equation

hepatic

homeostasis

homozygous

hyperopia

hypophysis

hypoxia

incus

isoenzyme

isotonic

ketosis

LH

lymph

macrophage

mast cells

menstrual cycle

metamorphosis

mineralocorticoid

morula

myelin

neuron

notochord

operon

osmosis

parasympathetic

parthenogenesis

peristalsis

photosynthesis

pituitary

plastid

poikilotherm

pons

proteostomate

purine

pyruvate

reflex arc

replication

Rh factor

saccule

sarcoplasm

secretin

skin glands

steroids

summation

surfactant

stroke volume

succession

sympatric speciation

synapse

systole

teleolecithal

telophase

test cross

tetanus

tetrad

thalamus

thymine

transcription

transformation

translation

triplet

trophic levels

trophoblast

trypsin

tubules

Turner's syndrome

uracil

utricle

vasomotor center

virus

vitamins

vitreous body

zygote

Chemistry Terms

absorption spectra

acetals

acid dissociation

aldehydes

aldol condensation

aliphatic carbons

alkanes

alkenes

alkynes

alloy

amides

amines

amino acids

amorphic

anion

anomer

aromatic compounds

Arrhenius equation

atomic mass

atomic number

atomic weight

Avogadro's number

azides

Bahmer series

benzene reactions

Bohr effect

Boyle's law

b.p. elevation

Bronsted-Lowery

Brown ring test

buffer systems

carbanion

carbohydrates

carbonium ion

carboxylic acids

catalyst

cation

cell potentials

Charles Law

chiral center

cis-trans

combustion

combined gas law

condensation

covalent bond

dehydration

Dalton's law

DeBrogle equation

dipole

disaccharides

diasteriomers

Dulong law

E1/E2 reactions

electrochemistry

electrophoresis

emission spectra

EMF

empirical formula

enantiomer

endothermic

enolization

enthalpy

epimer

epoxides

equilibrium

equivalent weight

esterification

esters

ethers

exothermic

Faraday's law

fatty acids

Fisher projections

formality

free fatty acids

freezing point

Gibbs free energy

glycerol

glycosidic linkage

Graham's law

Grignard reaction

half-cell reactions

halogenation

hemiacetal

Henderson-Hasselbach

Hess's law

Hund's law

hybridization

hydrogenation

hydrolysis

ideal gas law

ionization energy

isotope

kinetic energy

LeChatelier principle

Markownikoff's rule

molality

molecular formula

monosaccharides

Newman projections

nucleophilic

osmotic pressure

oxidation-reduction

periodic table

phase equilibria

pKa

polymorphic

polysaccharides

racemic mixtures

rate law

resolution

saponification

solubility product

specific gravity

STP

substitution reaction

titrations

Wolf-Kishner

indicators

isoelectric point

IUPAC names

kinetics

Lewis structures

meso compound

molarity

molecular geometry

Nernst equation

nitrification

optical activity

oxidation

oxidizing agents

Perfect gas law

phenols

Plank's constant

polypeptides

quantum number

Raolt's law

reducing agents

resonance

sigma bond

Sn1/Sn2 reactions

spontaneous reaction

stereoisomer

tautomerism

triglycerides

x-ray

ionic bonding

isomorphic

ketones

lactones

melting point

metallic bonding

mole

molecular weight

neutralization

normality

orbital

oxidation number

peptides

pH

pi body

polarity

proteins

radioactive decay

rate constant

reduction

ring strain

solubility

specific heat

stereochemistry

stoichemistry

thermodynamics

Vander Walls force

zwitterion

Physics Terms

AC circuits

alpha particles

angular momentum

batteries

beta particles

B.T.U.

cathode

centripetal force

conductors

converging lenses

critical temperature

decay constant

acceleration

ampere

anode

beats

binding energy

bulk modulus

Celsius

charge

conservation

Coulomb's law

current

decibel

adiabatic

amplitude

Archimede's law

Bernoulli's law

buoyant forces

capacitance

centrifugal force

conduction

convection

critical angle

DC circuits

density

dielectrics

diverging lenses

efficiency

electromagnetic force

equilibrium

focal length

frequency

fusion

half-life

heat of vaporization

horsepower

impedance

inertia

interface

isotope

k-capture

kinetic energy

loop theorem

mass

neutron

Ohm's law

Pascal's law

periodic motion

photon

planetary motion

point theorem

power

proton

real image

relativity

series circuit

static friction

sound waves

surface tension

tension

Toricelli's principle

translational motion

virtual image

voltage

watt

Young's modulus

diopter

Doppler effect

elasticity

electromotive force

farenheight

focal point

friction

gamma rays

harmonic motion

heat transfer

illumination

index of refraction

insulators

internal resistance

isothermal process

Kelvin

Kirchoff's law

magnetic field

mass deficit

Newton's laws

optics

pendulum

phase angle

pi meson

Plank's constant

positron

pressure

quantum mechanics

reflection

resistance

shear modulus

spectrum

stored energy

tensile strength

thermal expansion

torque

transverse waves

viscosity

voltmeter

wavelength

displacement

dyne

electric fields

electrostatics

fission

force

friction force

gravity

heat of fusion

Hooke's law

image distance

inductance

intensity

inverse square

joules

Kepler's law

longitudinal wave

magnification

mu meson

object distance

parallel circuit

period

photoelectric

pitch

point charge

potential energy

projectile motion

radiation

refraction

scalar

Snell's law

standing wave

superposition

tensile stress

thin lens formula

transistor

vector velocity

visible light spectrum

volume

work

The writers of the MCAT assume that you've had one year each of general biology, physics, inorganic chemistry, and organic chemistry. Most formulas, if needed, will be provided to you. It would be helpful, though, if you're at least familiar with the formulas, especially in chemistry and physics. Even if you aren't required to use a particular formula for direct computations, knowledge of those formulas might help you answer a question you might otherwise not be able to answer because you'll have a better understanding of what's being asked.

In some cases, your knowledge of formulas will help you derive answers more quickly. That could be important since the MCAT is a timed exam. No calculus is needed for any of the sections, but some math skills are definitely required. The following is a list of math skills expected of you or are important in being able to answer questions. Master them before attempting to take the exam.

1. General Algebra (sophomore high school level)
2. Understanding of exponents and logarithms
3. Knowledge of scientific notation
4. Interpretation of graphs, charts, and tables
5. Knowledge of trigonometric functions
6. Knowledge of metric units (and their English conversions)
7. Knowledge of percentage calculations
8. Understanding of statistical means and ranges
9. Understanding of significant numbers
10. Vector calculations (addition and subtraction)

In addition to the other suggestions, some good ways to prepare for the quantitative aspects of this section such as graph and tabular analysis are:

- When you read articles, don't just look at figures, graphs, charts, and tables in passing; analyze them. Spend time interpreting a graph's meaning and make sure you understand what it's showing you. Before long, you'll automatically look at figure or table and interpret it more readily.

- Get in the habit of looking at how the axes are labeled as soon as you look at the graph. On the MCAT, questions can easily be missed because a graph is labeled in grams, for example, but the question may require an answer in kilograms. Be careful.

- Take a statistics course. There will be questions that require you to look at a collection of research data and derive answers from it. A knowledge of statistics can improve your chances of answering questions more easily and with more speed and confidence. An added benefit is that medical schools look favorably on a transcript which includes statistics, since knowledge of statistics is important in interpreting scientific data and medical results.

- Don't limit yourself to certain types of quantitative data. Be as comfortable with a graph of medical data as you are with a graph of astrophysics data.

Preparation for the Verbal Reasoning Section of the MCAT

This section is designed to measure your ability to read passages and evaluate information presented in them. If you've been reading all along, then you're probably ahead on this one. If you aren't a daily reader, and you don't evaluate and/or analyze the information you read, then you need to start doing that now. Here are some tips that will help you improve your reading speed and comprehension specifically for the kinds of readings you'll see on the MCAT.

- Read 4 or 5 short articles every day (500 to 600 words in length). This is about the length of the passages on the exam and will get you accustomed to reading several short articles at one sitting. Try to read the articles one after another so that you develop the habit of leaving one set of ideas and starting on a different set of ideas right away without any mental interruptions. This is what you'll be expected to do on the MCAT.

- Read a variety of subjects each day, not just one topic which you happen to enjoy reading about. For example, when you sit down to read, read about the humanities, the social sciences, economics, history, anthropology, science, etc. Become a "diverse" reader and learn about different things. You'll also have an advantage over other students who haven't trained themselves to read about diverse subjects.

- Subscribe to several magazines (or find them at the library) which contain a number of varied topics. Newsweek, Time, U.S. News and World Report are good ones. Reading various topics in these well-written magazines exposes you to ideas that are favorite subjects on the verbal reasoning part of the MCAT and also exposes you to a variety of different writing styles. Furthermore, by becoming conversant with different topics, you won't be shocked during the MCAT when you have to read and interpret an article on the fiscal and protectionist policies of the industrial world followed by an article about the mating habits of South American spiders.

- When doing a practice MCAT test, try reading the questions first before reading the passage. This may help you identify critical information as you're reading. Underline important words and phrases, and don't be afraid to make notes in the margins. These will serve as landmarks that help you locate pertinent details and key ideas.

Preparing for the Writing Sample

Naturally, the best way to prepare for the writing section is to take a writing course designed to teach you how to organize central ideas and write in a coherent and logical manner. Medical schools want students who have good communication skills, both oral and written, since doctors must be able to communicate effectively.

There's really no one good way to prepare for the writing section if you're not familiar with the basics of writing. One student who had taken the exam told me that he prepared himself by reading a passage from a magazine, then writing about it for 30 minutes. When he came to the essay part of the MCAT, he breezed right through it. This is why you need to make room in your undergraduate curriculum for courses that improve writing skills or ones that force you to write. Here are some suggestions that should help you when you're actually taking the test:

- As you read the essay topic carefully, underline key words and ideas so that you can quickly go back to them when needed. Utilize your 30 minutes per question wisely by spending no more than 5 minutes thinking and planning what you're going to write, 20 minutes actually writing the essay, and 5 minutes proofreading and rewriting if necessary.

- If there's more than one idea, question, or concept within the topic, make a note of them by placing a check or number next to them. Be sure to address "all" the topics mentioned, since they're mentioned for a reason and not just placed there as fillers. Look at the question and pay attention to any clues you can use to organize your essay. You need to write your essay in a way that will fulfill any requirements given. Think in terms of answering the question by either analyzing, explaining, discussing, summarizing, tracing, etc.

- Sit and think about what you've read for several minutes and reread if necessary. Focus on the key ingredients of your essay:

  - the central idea, i.e. what the essay means in plain terms

- the issues that the essay topic and essay question want you to address

- the key points that must be emphasized in your essay

- When writing the essay, divide it into 3 main parts as follows:

  1. An explanation of what the essay topic means. Always begin by writing an introductory sentence that explains the topic, followed by your position. The introductory sentence should also give the reader an idea of what will follow. Doing this demonstrates your understanding of the written material.

  2. Incorporation of your ideas into the main theme and concepts of the essay topic. This includes addressing all the critical issues and questions required of you.

  3. A conclusion that brings together and summarizes what you've written about or gives an alternative view or hypothesis.

- Don't try to write as much as you can at the expense of quality. Place more emphasis on making sure the essay is written clearly and logically rather than on number of words in the essay. Also, watch for grammar, punctuation, spelling, etc. Intersperse long with short sentences, use active versus passive verbs, and smooth out the flow of the essay by beginning your sentences with phrases and transitional words rather than using "The" all the time. Remember, the purpose of the essay is to write in direct prose, not in jargon or journal style.

- Don't be sloppy. Try to write as clearly and legibly as possible so that the person reading your essay understands what you're trying to communicate. I've read many exam answers written by good college students who were so sloppy that I couldn't understand their answers. In my case, I just mark them wrong. Because the essay is considered an important part of the MCAT, take it seriously and do the best work you can.

To give you an idea of what exactly the readers of the writing sample are looking for when scoring your answers, here are the criteria for the scoring system. Essays are scored 1 to 6, then converted to a letter score from J (the lowest) to T (the highest). The three criteria used to judge the writing are thoroughness, depth, and clarity of ideas presented in the essay. If the scorers differ by more than one point, a third reader determines the total score for the paper.

1 J - K: None of the writing criteria were addressed. There were marked problems with organization and mechanics that make the language very difficult to follow.

2 L - M: There were serious problems with one or more of the writing criteria. There were also problems with organization and analysis of the topic and recurrent mechanical errors, resulting in language that is occasionally difficult to follow.

3 N - O: Neglects or distorts one of more of the writing criteria or presents only a minimal treatment of the topic. There is some clarity of thought, but it may be simplistic. There are problems in organization, although the essay demonstrates a basic control of vocabulary and sentence structure. The language, however, may not effectively communicate the writer's ideas.

4 P - Q: There is a moderate treatment of the three writing criteria. The essay shows clarity of thought but it may lack complexity. There is a demonstration of coherent organization, though some digressions are evident. The writing shows an overall control of vocabulary and sentence structure.

5 R - S: There is substantial treatment of all writing criteria. The essay shows some depth of thought, coherent organization, and control of vocabulary and sentence structure.

6 T: There is thorough treatment of all three writing criteria. The essay shows depth and complexity of thought, focused and coherent organization, and a superior control of vocabulary and sentence structure.

Some Final Hints for the MCAT

- If you can afford it, and think you really need it, look into the possibility of taking one of the professional MCAT preparatory courses. Even though all the information you'll need for the MCAT is included in your introductory college courses, the critical thinking and analysis required on the new MCAT is unlike anything you may be used to. Furthermore, these courses do an especially good job in reviewing the science topics covered on the exam.

- Try to spend at least three, and preferably six, months preparing for the MCAT. If it has been a while since your last chemistry or physics course, it's especially important that you review at length.

- When you study, never study for more than an hour at a time. Take a ten minute break before going back to your books or notes. Studies have shown that most people, whether they realize it or not, rapidly lose concentration and the ability to absorb information after only one hour of study. Taking a short break periodically will reset your mind and your attitude for another session of studying.

- A few weeks before the MCAT, train yourself to go to bed at a reasonable hour and wake up at the same time you'll be waking up for the exam. This conditioning program is important for proper relaxation. It's well known that test anxiety during a long exam is more difficult to cope with when the individual is fatigued. If you have to, learn a relaxation technique and use it before the exam.

- Don't study the night before the exam. Relax and try not to think about the next day.

- Get plenty of rest the day before so that you'll wake up refreshed and feeling well rested.

- Eat a light breakfast. There's a 10 minute break during the morning session, at which time you can eat a snack you brought if you're hungry.

- Don't eat a heavy lunch. After the morning session, the last thing you need is to become sluggish for the afternoon writing and biological sciences sections. There's also a 10 minute break during the afternoon session, at which time you can get a quick snack.

- Make sure you're at the test center well beforehand, since you won't be allowed to come in once the exam has begun.

- If you have a special request for testing accommodations due to disabilities etc., make sure the MCAT Program Office receives them no later than the late registration receipt deadline.

   If your preparation has been an ongoing process, you'll do much better than if you try to utilize these techniques a few months or even a few weeks before the exam. It's never too late to start, though. Begin now and be very conscientious about your preparation. A few months of hard work are much better than none at all.

8

Medical School Interview

If a medical school feels that your initial qualifications make you a good candidate for medical school, it will then grant you an interview. Almost all medical schools require an interview, since acceptances are not granted without one. If you're fortunate enough to be awarded an interview, you can be sure that the medical school is interested enough to find out more about you.

This is a good opportunity for medical schools to question you about your application, any items on your autobiographical sketch, or any discrepancies in your grades or MCAT scores. This is also a good way for medical schools to screen out what they see as psychological misfits who may not be well suited for life as medical students or as future doctors. Most of all, the interview is a good way for a medical school to see what you're like as a person and how well you respond and communicate.

Based on a survey of admissions officers, it was found that many schools regard the interview as one of the more important criteria in judging a potential candidate. It was surprising that some of the respondents considered the interview even more important than MCAT scores and letters of recommendations from undergraduate schools. In general, the admissions interviewers said they needed to identify the following combination of factors during the interview process. Before going on an interview, candidates should make sure their credentials include them.

- Maturity and motivation for medicine.
- Ability to succeed.
- Interpersonal skills and communicative abilities.
- Ability to evaluate medicine as a career in relation to a student's strengths and weaknesses.
- Academic ability to withstand the rigors of a medical education.
- Common sense or lack thereof.
- Experiences that provide a broad perspective.
- Ability to endure the academic and social stresses of medical school.
- Intellectual curiosity reflecting a love of learning.
- Humanitarianism or concern for others.
- Adaptability and flexibility

How to Prepare for an Interview

The first rule of thumb for medical school interviews is to present yourself in an open and honest manner without trying to "psych out" the interviewer. In other words, don't think that you can go on an interview, tell the interviewer exactly what he or she wants to hear, and come out looking like a winner. Each medical school interviews its applicants differently and, therefore, what you might expect at one medical school will be completely opposite of what you'll actually encounter. Because of the varied nature of medical school interviews, it's to your advantage to write or phone the admissions office before your interview and get complete information about the following:

1. Is the interview conducted by one person or is it a group interview?

2. What's the normal length of time for the interview?

3. What kind of individuals make up the interview committee?

4. Are the interviewers doctors? Are they researchers?

5. In what kind of setting will the interview be conducted?

It's very helpful to read the school's catalogue a few days beforehand to get an idea of curriculums, programs, activities, etc. Knowing the right information about a prospective medical school is important when an interviewer wants to discuss why you applied to that particular school. It's no different than a prospective employer asking you what it is about the company that makes you think you'd want to work there. Anticipating questions can also help you prepare by making you feel more comfortable and relaxed. A long list of actual medical school interview questions is included in this chapter.

I recently spoke to an admissions committee member who had just finished interviewing prospective students for several months. I asked him about the kinds of things he looked for when interviewing so many different types of well-qualified applicants. He broke his system down into five areas. Naturally, each interviewer is different and looks for certain qualities when judging applicants. These five areas, however, can give you a good indication of what many admissions committee members think are important characteristics in medical school applicants.

A. *Hands on experience in a clinical setting:* Did the student work in an emergency room, as a candy striper, or with a doctor, since all of these contribute to a more realistic understanding of medicine? In other words, was the student exposed to the realities and rigors of medicine before deciding to make a career of it?

B. *Knowledge of the profession:* Does the student have some knowledge of different specialties and what it really takes to be a physician? Is he or she aware of the profession through some sort of practical experience?

C. *Length of time interested in medicine:* Is this something the student has been interested in for a long time or just recently? If it has been a long-term goal, what kinds of things were done to accomplish that goal?

D. *Personality:* Does the student have the ability to communicate about himself or herself? Can he or she talk about relationships? Does he or she have an experience in communication either in public or elsewhere?

E. *Role Model:* Is there someone in the family close to the student who has served as a role model and encouraged medicine as a career? This can be derived from area A.

Interviewing Minority Students

Although the issue of minority status has no place in the interview process, minority students have to be aware of problems that could affect their performance on the interview. Unfortunately for the minority student, the majority of medical school interviewers will be non-minority individuals who may have preconceived notions that could be hard to handle. Fortunately, though, there are record numbers of minority students being accepted to medical schools and are doing very well.

If you're a minority student and you encounter an interviewer whose remarks seem to be insulting or insensitive, the last thing you want to do is become angry or confrontational. Becoming angry will adversely affect your interview conduct and make you more ill at ease and overly anxious during the rest of the interview process. Rather than becoming angry, help the interviewer understand the reasons for your past experiences, deficiencies, and activities. Use your background to show your accomplishments and to demonstrate how you were able to overcome difficult life situations and get where you are today. If after being interviewed, you feel that you were treated unfairly, don't hesitate to write to the admissions officer and describe in detail your reasons for feeling the way you do.

Interview Questions

The following is a list of actual medical school interview questions I've compiled over the years from faculty members, interviewers, and medical students. The advantage of having so many questions at your disposal is twofold. Firstly, it helps you anticipate the most frequently asked questions so that you can appear confident and poised. Secondly, it will give you a chance to formulate some new opinions and eliminate your weak points as you read through some of the questions.

You'll be surprised at some of the odd questions asked by interviewers, and it's certainly better to be prepared now than to be shocked or surprised at the interview itself. By studying the questions, you can get an insight into the kinds of things admissions committees feel are important for medical school applicants to at least be thinking about.

Frequently Asked Questions

What do you think about the quality of today's health care system?

What kinds of books do you like to read?

Do you watch news on TV or read the newspaper to keep up with current events?

What qualities do you have that would make you a good physician?

What negative qualities do you have that may be a problem to you as a doctor?

Tell me about your childhood.

What are / were your interests and hobbies?

What are your alternate plans should you not be accepted to medical school?

Tell me about yourself.

Have you thought about a specialty after getting an M.D.?

Tell me about the organizations you belong to.

Why do you think your MCAT scores are lower than your grades reflect they should be?

Why are your grades lower than your MCAT scores reflect they should be?

How do you feel about socialized medicine?

Why did you choose this medical school to apply to?

What kinds of people do you like to surround yourself with?

How did you first become interested in becoming a doctor?

What is the most attractive aspect of medicine for you?

How does your family feel about you going to medical school?

How will you support yourself while in medical school?

Do you think you'll be able to be successful in medical school and maintain a healthy family life? How?

Do you have any idea what a doctor's life is like?

Why should we choose you among all the other applicants?

What do you think is the major problem in today's health care system?

How would you handle a terminally ill patient?

Tell me about your hospital experiences.

Tell me about your work while in college.

Discuss some of the factors that led up to your decision to become a doctor.

Tell me about your family's background.

What do like about this school in particular?

Tell me about your high school activities.

How does your family feel about your being a doctor?

Tell me about your parents.

What kind of relationship do you have with your parents?

How did your hospital experience relate to your decision to apply to medical school?

Tell me about your brothers and sisters.

Tell me something about your outside reading interests.

What are the negative aspects of being a doctor?

What is your most unique quality?

Do you enjoy being challenged?

How well do you cope with emergency situations?

How do you think your weaknesses will affect you as a medical student?

Do you think your strengths will help you through medical school?

What are some past experiences that you feel will help you as a doctor?

How do you spend your spare time with your family?

Do you think medical school affects family relationships? If so how would you overcome that?

What do you think you can offer this incoming class that other applicants can't?

How much do you keep up with current events?

What do you see wrong with the medical profession?

How do you see yourself?

How do others see you?

Give a brief review of your research.

More Interview Questions

How do you think the health care system will change in the years ahead?

What factors will play a role in molding our decisions on extension of life?

What's the most recent book you've read and what was it about?

Who are your favorite writers?

What kinds of magazines do you read?

Who are your state senators?

How can you be an effective doctor if you admit to having negative qualities?

What kinds of childhood activities did you participate in?

How did you manage going to school and having a family?

Do you and your wife find it difficult during the school year?

How did you feel about Desert Storm?

Why did you select the individuals you did to write letters for you?

What did you do in the military?

What kinds of music do you enjoy listening to?

How do you think society should curb the rising cost of medical care?

What do you think of the admissions process of medical school?

Do you think the admissions process is fair?

Where do you see yourself in 10 to 15 years?

What was your worst course in college?

What's the one question you don't want to be asked on this interview?

How would you affect the health care system?

Do you like to teach?

How would you feel about teaching at a medical college?

What subject did you enjoy most in college? Why?

What is the greatest medical problem facing us today?

Do you think medical school will be fun? Why or why not?

Give two adjectives that best describe you.

Would you be interested in participating in medical associations?

How do handle people who come to you with problems?

Would you be interested in practicing in underprivileged or back country areas?

How would you handle a seductive patient?

How would you handle a drunk patient?

Suppose you had your ideal practice 20 years from now. Describe it.

Did your parents or anyone else push you into medicine?

As a woman, how would you deal with having a family and a medical career?

How would your patients describe you?

Tell me how you feel about medical ethics in today's society?

Why did you go to graduate school instead of medical school?

Do you think you might like to do research as a doctor?

How would you handle a discussion with the family of a dying patient?

How would you deal with a terminally ill patient who refused to take his medicine?

Why do you want to be a doctor instead of a nurse?

What are your feelings about euthanasia?

What do you do for fun?

Trace the development of your interest in medicine, correlating it with your college experiences.

Who influenced your decision about medical school the most?

Explain your summer internships and/or activities.

Tell me about your independent studies.

Why did you choose this geographical area?

Tell me about your research activities.

How can you integrate family life into a medical career?

Do you think high school activities are important in medical school evaluations?

If you had a young patient who was on dialysis and wanted to discontinue treatment, what would you do?

How did you manage to keep up your grades and be in athletics?

What makes you so certain you can handle medical school?

Why do you think that you would want to see sick people all day?

Does death bother you very much?

Do you feel that a doctor should become hardened to death?

How do you feel about working around patients with contagious diseases?

Do you feel that a doctor should be involved in community affairs?

What kind of social life do you think doctors have?

What kinds of sports are you interested in?

What do you think about public television? The arts?

How would you deal with a patient who refused to pay you?

How would you deal with a regular patient who had poor sanitary habits?

Do you think your extracurricular activities helped you prepare for medical school?

How do you think your major will help you in medicine?

How well do you think you'll do in medical school if you only got Bs in college chemistry?

Why did you attend the college you did?

How much time do you spend studying?

What do you think about computers?

How do you feel about the use of computers in the medical field?

Do you think that computers will become or are already indispensable in medicine?

How would you decide which medical school to attend?

Do you want to get into medicine for prestige and money?

Would you remain a physician if we had socialized medicine? Why or why not?

Do you think that liberal arts courses are important? Why or why not?

Why were your grades lower during your freshman year than they were during your remaining years?

Would you change any part of your college life if you could?

What kinds of alternate career choices do you have?

Do you like qualitative or quantitative science?

Describe the perfect physician.

How would you react to a patient who insists on another doctor?

Would you tell a patient to get a second opinion if you were sure of your diagnosis?

How do you feel about the rising cost of malpractice insurance?

Is there anything we can do to keep malpractice costs down?

How would you handle a colleague you knew was taking drugs?

How much confidence do you have in yourself?

Would you consider a foreign medical school?

Do you help your wife around the house?

Describe the ideal medical student.

Do you think the best students make the best doctors?

Why is there a drug abuse problem in the medical profession?

Do you know what the divorce rate is among physicians?

How will you handle the stress of being a doctor?

How can the drug and alcohol problem among health professionals be alleviated?

Why do you think people are losing confidence in doctors?

How was it being raised in a large family?

What would you do if you suspected child abuse?

Would you react to child abuse in the same way if the victim was the child of a friend?

Do you think a doctor should ignore his or her feelings when dealing with patients?

Do you think that making life and death decisions makes a doctor callous?

Have modern doctors lost that human touch with their patients?

What do you think patients look for in a physician?

Have you ever been exposed to real life trauma?

Do you think that every student should experience the tragedy of death and disease before deciding on medicine?

Why is your GPA so low?

Don't you think it'll be harder for you to maintain your grades in medical school?

What will you have to do in order to be successful in medical school?

Do you think that MCAT scores reflect how a person will do in medical school?

Have you thought about serving in the armed forces after medical school?

What was it like traveling around Europe?

What kinds of questions did you expect to be asked before you came here?

Do you think doctors should do much outside reading?

Do you think today's doctors are as compassionate as they used to be? Why or why not?

As medical technology advances, how will doctors maintain a personal relationship with their patients?

How would you handle a patient who just had a miscarriage and can't have any more children?

How demanding would you be with your nursing staff?

What are your thoughts about the growing number of hospice programs?

Do you think more doctors should become involved in programs like hospice?

Which school activities did you enjoy most? Why?

How much of your college expenses did you pay for yourself?

If you started college over, would you change your major? Why or why not?

Why was your class standing so low?

Would you rather work independently or as part of a team? Why?

What type of person do you enjoy working for?

How many times have you changed your college major? Why did you finally settle on this one?

What courses gave you the most trouble?

Would you be willing to practice medicine wherever you were needed in return for a scholarship?

What do you think about organized religion?

Would you rather watch or participate in sports?

Do you get along well with your boss?

Do you think there should be a minimum GPA for entrance to medical school?

What can this medical school offer you that the others can't?

How can I be of help to you during this interview?

What are your feelings about routine work?

How did like moving with your family as a child?

Do you feel that living in many places was an advantage? Why or why not?

Which one of your jobs did you enjoy the most? The Least? Why?

Would you change anything about your childhood?

Do you think interviews are important? Why or why not?

What would you do if, during your senior year of medical school, you decided that medicine was not for you?

Is there anything about medicine that would make you give it up?

What qualities do you look for in your friends?

Give me an example of the perfect job for you.

How much emphasis should we place on your MCAT scores?

What was the hardest year of college for you? Why?

Do you think a science major is important for medical students to have? Why or why not?

How would you handle a patient you suspected was psychosomatic?

Is intellectual fulfillment one of the main reasons you chose medicine?

Do you think the medical profession needs more researchers and less practitioners?

How do you feel about the growing number of specialists?

How would you compare our system of medicine with that of other countries?

Can we learn anything from foreign medical systems?

What do you think the unique qualities of this school are?

Have you read any journal articles lately? Tell me about it.

What have you learned from some of your readings?

How can a physician possibly keep up with all the scientific information available?

Did you enjoy doing research

Why didn't you pursue a graduate degree?

With all the work you'll have to do, how will you devote any time to your wife and family?

Why on earth do you want to get into this business?

What would you like to get most out of your medical training?

How do think being female will affect you in medical school?

Should dealing with a terminally ill child be any different than dealing with an adult?

Do you really know what's involved in going to medical school?

Do you try to keep up with current events?

Why did you major in English?

Do you think the attitude of the patient is important in the healing process?

How much can a doctor affect a patient's attitude?

Are you the type of person others come to for help?

Tell me about your orchestra experience.

If you changed your major before, why do you think you won't change your mind again?

What factors would alter your decision concerning the extension of life?

Do you think it's in our best interests to extend life?

What are your feelings about performing an abortion on a 13 year old?

What are your feelings about abortion when the fetus is severely retarded?

Should doctors be willing to be evaluated by their peers? Why or why not?

Should we believe your grades or your MCAT scores? Why?

How well do you know the individuals who wrote letters for you?

Do you think letters are a good source of information for admissions committees?

Did any of your military experience help you in deciding on medical school?

Do you think the military made you more mature and better able to know what you want to do?

Are you a self-motivated individual?

How is your relationship with your brothers and sisters?

What do your brothers and sisters do for a living?

What quality is most important for a doctor to have?

Why did you wait so long before going to college?

Do you think that starting college later was an advantage?

With your background, why didn't you apply to vet school?

Why did you participate in the activities you did?

How would describe the ideal medical practice?

What happened during your third year that affected your grades so much?

Do you think athletics was the cause of your poor grades the first year?

Did you apply to this school because of its name?

Do you consider yourself intelligent or did you have to work hard for your grades?

What have you learned from your research experience?

What have you learned from your hospital experience?

What did you get most out of your extracurricular activities?

Is there one memory of school that stands out more than the rest?

Should personality be an important factor in the admissions process?

Is there a certain personality type that doctors should have?

What type of supervisor would you be?

Are you an introvert or an extrovert? Would that have an impact on you as a doctor?

How would you convince a terminally ill patient to continue treatment if it were very painful?

How would you react to a young patient who wanted to be sterilized?

Give me two reasons why you would not want to be a doctor?

Will you reapply to medical school if you're not accepted?

Would you consider dental school if you're not accepted into medical school?

What's the biggest contribution medicine has made this decade?

How do you think medical advances are affecting the individual patient?

Will there be a time when a doctor is nothing more than a technician?

What will you enjoy most about medical school?

What will you enjoy least about medical school?

Describe yourself twenty years from now.

What kinds of news events have you found interesting lately?

Are you interested in world affairs? Why or why not?

Do you find it difficult studying for long periods of time?

Do you know any doctors personally who may have stimulated your interest in medicine?

What did you get most out of your four years of college?

Is there anything you really disliked about college in general?

Have you been involved in extracurricular activities throughout your entire 4 years of college?

How do you react to stress and pressure?

Many questions are asked about things students include in their autobiographical sketches. Make sure you're well prepared to answer detailed questions concerning anything you include in that part of your application. If you wrote it, it's fair game, so be honest about your background. Also, be prepared to discuss topics currently in the news. Some frequently discussed topics you should prepare for and feel comfortable talking about include:

- Today's social issues

- Current news events

- Discussions about family

- Reasons for wanting to become a doctor

- Modern health care issues such as pros and cons of HMOs, rising health care costs, etc.

- Controversial issues such as abortion, birth control, euthanasia, life extension, etc.

- Discussions about your past experiences

- Discussions about anything on your autobiographical sketch

I recently spoke to a medical school professor right after he completed an interview with an applicant. He'd told me that he gave the student a negative rating based on the student's answer to one simple question. The interviewer wanted to know how long the student had a desire to be a doctor. Apparently, the student's desire wasn't sincere enough as far as the interviewer was concerned. The student mentioned that one of his fraternity brothers told him that his grades were good enough to get into medical school and that he should try to make it as a doctor. Dumb advice! In the interviewer's opinion, the student didn't put much thought into his decision and, therefore, wasn't sincere in his desire to become a doctor.

Be careful about making dumb comments such as this during the stress of an interview. Sometimes the pressure will make you say things you really don't mean or shouldn't say. The best way to get through any interview successfully is to be honest, be yourself, and try to anticipate as many questions as you can in order to be prepared. Take advantage of all the help you can get, because one question can mean the difference between acceptance and rejection.

The same interviewer also told me that the two traits most interviewers look for in applicants are confidence and poise. In order to ensure a good impression, you need to act confident and maintain your composure even when you don't know the answer to a question or feel uncomfortable answering it. Often, the confidence you show in yourself when you can't answer a question will mean more than the confidence you exude when answering a question anyone can answer. So remember to be HEP - Honest, Extroverted, and Poised at all times, regardless of the questions being asked.

What students don't realize is that most interviewers care little about right or wrong answers. What they're really looking for are statements that are well thought out, expressive, and show good communicative skills. An interviewer, for example, won't care what your personal views are on abortion or socialized medicine; what he or she cares about is how you express your own personal opinion, no matter what that opinion is, and whether it's totally in opposition to anyone else's.

A friend of mine told me that one of his favorite questions to ask is "Tell me something about your mom." He feels that, since moms are a good subject of conversation, anyone with good communicative skills and good thought processes should be able to answer that one well. After all, who doesn't have strong opinions, one way or another, about their moms? Here's how two candidates responded to that same question.

A. "Well, you know; she's good old mom. What can I say about my mother except that she's a great person and I love her. Without her, I guess I wouldn't be where I am today."

B. "My mother is a wonderful, caring, and humorous person. I don't think that I would be the person I am if it weren't for her. While I was growing up, she was always a strict parent and made sure that we did very well in school. But even though she was pretty strict, I remember always laughing at some of the funny remarks she would make to us children. Whenever we were sick or upset about something, her humor always picked us up. Even now, we can count on her to cheer us up. My mom never worked - she was always home with us because she felt that her job was raising her kids. She never regretted that. I guess of all the qualities that describe her, the best one would be her devotion to her family. And her devotion to me and my brothers and sisters is something I'll remember for the rest of my life."

I don't have to tell you which answer the interviewer was more impressed with. Quite honestly, he thought the first candidate was a lousy interviewee, whereas the second was absolutely great. Even if the first candidate would have had negative remarks about his mother, it would have been better than the short, somewhat thoughtless answer he gave.

The lesson here is that you need to say something substantial, even if you have some negative feelings. Of course, you should dampen your negative feelings a little so that you don't sound too cynical or bitter. Most importantly, though, say something that will make the interviewer feel that you're thinking about what you're saying.

Many times, interviewers want to see if candidates are aware of the expectations imposed on the medical profession. The following list of expectations was taken from an issue of *Medical Education* and should be read several times before an interview. Knowing these will help you seem more informed about your future medical career. You may even want to use some of these expressions word for word during the interview whenever appropriate.

1. The doctor should be able to develop an effective relationship with his or her patients by:

- Having cultural, social, and religious sensitivity

- Taking a long-term supportive role in patient care

- Being sensitive, sympathetic, and equalitarian

- Developing effective communication

- Sharing information and involving patients

- Coping with close contact and emotional demands

2. The doctor should demonstrate technical competence by:

- Intervening to affect a cure where possible

- Keeping up to date with developments in health care

- Being flexible and receptive to new medical ideas

- Learning to cope with uncertainties and limitations

- Understanding the process of decision-making

- Managing emotional and psychological problems

3. The doctor should demonstrate professional responsibility by:

- Critical evaluation of his or her own performance

- Learning to judge and be judged through peer review

- Accepting the challenge of continuing education

- Maintaining the highest quality health care

- Contributing to the development of health policy

4. The doctor should demonstrate social responsibility by:

- Containing the high costs of health care

- Playing a role in health education and prevention

- Suggesting equitable and cost-effective health care

5. The doctor should demonstrate economic responsibility by:

- Recognizing the economic side of clinical decisions

- Basing management decisions on cost/benefit factors

- Critically appraising efficiency in health care

- Using expensive technology wisely

- Rationing services according to need priority

- Developing moral, technical, and social guidelines for resources

- Developing guidelines for priority identification

6. The doctor should be able to arrange an optimum patient care environment in order to:

- Ensure accessibility to patients
- Work as an effective member of the health care team
- Conduct research in order to improve health care

The last page of this chapter includes an example of the kind of interview evaluation sheet that interviewers at some medical school fill out after interviewing an applicant. Read the interviewer's written comments. They may be helpful in letting you see how that particular interviewer felt about certain traits and characteristics.

Selling Yourself on the Interview

An interview is really your opportunity to sell yourself to the interviewer. According to many experts, there are four main ways of selling yourself: (1) Enthusiasm, (2) Sincerity, (3) Tactfulness, and (4) Courtesy.

Enthusiasm is the interest you take in the interview itself and the positive manner in which you act towards the interviewer when he or she asks questions or discusses issues. One of the best ways to show enthusiasm is to ask some questions. So before the interview, study the medical school's catalogue and have some questions prepared before you go.

Sincerity is synonymous with honesty. A trained interviewer can spot dishonesty and phony answers and will give you a negative evaluation because of it. I certainly would. If you don't know the answer to a question, don't make one up; be honest enough to admit that you don't know. I personally think character *does* matter, and I place honesty and sincerity very high on my list of characteristics.

Tactfulness is important in answering questions that require you to disagree with the interviewer. For the most part, interviewers are pretty agreeable, but there will be some who love to put you on the spot. For example, if you have strong beliefs about abortion or socialized medicine, and the interviewer presses you about why you don't go along with the views of most doctors, don't get belligerent; just begin your answer with a simple, "I can understand why you would feel that way, and I respect your opinion on the matter, but I feel . . ."

Courtesy, or the lack of it, can literally kill the interview before it even gets going. Regardless of the question asked or the comments made, always be as courteous as possible throughout the entire interview. Not only will it make the interview more pleasant, it will leave a lasting impression on the interviewer when he or she is writing down comments right afterwards.

Selling yourself on the interview can be fairly easy as long as you understand what the interviewing committee members are looking for and you prepare yourself beforehand. Besides the suggestions already mentioned, here are a few key points that should help you sell yourself and seal the interview:

1. Prepare to discuss your handicaps and weaknesses. Don't be so naive as to think that your records don't show a weakness or two. Nearly everyone has something negative in their background, and your job is to recognize it and be able to discuss it directly and confidently. You may get an interviewer who will spend more time trying to flush out your weaknesses than your strengths. It's more difficult discussing the negatives about yourself. It's also more impressive watching someone talk about their weaknesses with finesse and agility. Always try to turn your weaknesses into strengths, or explain how you can improve or have improved upon those weaknesses.

2. Help the interviewer get at the right information. If you have special skills, experiences, and/or accomplish-ments that are important but aren't being discussed, be on the lookout for openings to highlight some of your achievements. Don't assume that everyone is a good interviewer and will ask the right questions.

3. Research everything you possibly can about the medical school at which you're being interviewed. Interviewers are always impressed by an applicant who has done his or her homework about their institution. Conversely, they aren't very tolerant of

applicants who don't know much about the place they've come for what may be the most important interview of their life. This could be a real blow to your chances. Therefore, know the school, be able to explain why you're interested in it, be familiar with what the school can offer you, and be able to discuss why you in particular would fit into their program.

4. Say only what needs to be said. Always stay on the subject and don't begin rambling about things that are unnecessary just for the sake of talking. You can avoid this problem by preparing and practicing some of the important frequently asked questions you could encounter during the interview.

5. Always prepare at least 5 questions to ask at the end of the interview. Normally, an interviewer will ask if you have any questions. Never say no! Ask one or two, but have five ready in case some have already been answered during the course of the interview. Asking questions will show interest and intelligence and is a good way to leave an impression with the interviewer.

6. Send a thank you note to the interviewer (you should know his or her name) as soon after the interview as possible. This will reinforce his or her recollection of you and will demonstrate that you're interested and that you're courteous. Be brief in your note and don't try to make excuses for a bad answer.

How to Dress for Interview Success

Any professional interviewer will tell you that the way you dress for an interview is one of the more important aspects of the interview process, since first impressions are formed even before you open your mouth. Therefore, to start off on the right foot, you need to dress to your advantage. For medical school interviews, this means following a few rules that will ensure giving a good impression.

Always dress conservatively. Medical school interviewers are professionals, and feel most comfortable talking to someone who also appears professional. Besides, what kind of statement would you send if you cared so little about your interview that you couldn't even dress decently? A suit and tie is a must for men; a dress is a must for women. Good colors to wear are blue, gray, black, brown, or dark green. Avoid bright flashy colors, loud ties, baggy or tight clothes, and casual attire. Remember, it's easier for a more liberal interviewer to accept a conservative interviewee than it is for a conservative interviewer to accept someone dressed as if it were an afterthought.

Interview Conduct

Normally, a medical school interview is very informal and relaxed. Some interviewers even like to make it a fun experience. There may be one or more interviewers present, but the atmosphere is usually cordial, and every effort is made to make you feel at ease. Interviewers are interested in your answers, but they're also interested in the way you handle yourself when asked questions about personal or controversial issues.

Forget about thinking up a "right" answer and just relax. The best way to act is to be yourself, since an admissions committee has the experience to see right through any facade and get a bad impression of your character. The following are some things to do and not to do during an interview.

Things To Do

Do make eye contact.
Do smile occasionally.
Do present a calm and self-assured appearance.
Do speak with a firm but gentle voice.
Do arrive early for the interview.
Do exhibit enthusiasm and sincerity.

Do show interest in the interview and the interviewer.

Do be courteous

Do listen carefully to the interviewer's question.

Do be honest if you don't know the answer to a particular question.

Do be prepared for general questions such as, "Tell me about yourself."

Do be yourself and always act natural.

Do dress appropriately and conservatively.

Do present a neat and clean appearance.

Do ask a question if there's a pause of silence.

Do thank the interviewer at the end of the interview (this is important).

Things Not To Do

Don't wring your hands.

Don't sit on the edge of your seat.

Don't fidget in your seat.

Don't put your hands near your face or mouth, especially when talking.

Don't use excessive hand motions.

Don't speak too loudly.

Don't mumble or make the interviewer repeat a question.

Don't get nervous when asked questions you're not familiar with.

Don't be afraid to ask for clarification to give you time to think.

Don't worry about thinking for a few seconds before answering a question.

Don't chew gum or smoke, even when offered.

Don't be flamboyant, overly zealous, or overbearing.

Don't respond to a serious question with a joke.

Don't correct an interviewer.

Don't look away when giving an answer or asking a question.

Don't criticize former employers, teachers, etc.

Don't use poor grammar

Don't be passive.

Don't lie!

9

Minority Admissions

Compared with years past, there's been a positive change in the proportion of minority students entering U.S. medical schools. Prior to 1968, most admissions committees sat back passively and waited to see what kinds of students would apply. Since then, however, there's been a dramatic shift not only in the composition of the applicant pool but also in the way students are recruited in order to diversify medical school student bodies.

Today, individuals who had never before considered entering medical school have been actively encouraged to apply. At the same time, programs have been established which assist minority students get the help they need in becoming competitive medical school candidates.

Minority Application, Acceptance, and Graduation Trends

During this decade, the total number of minority students applying to medical schools has decreased, but the overall acceptance rate has remained relatively stable. For example, during the 1997-98 school year, the percent of African Americans applicants accepted to medical schools was 38 percent compared with 36 percent in 1996 and 39 percent in 1995. The problem is that the percentage of minorities practicing medicine is less than half their representation in the general population. Not only has the AAMC's goal of increasing enrollments of minorities to reflect the growing diversity of the United States population not been met, there are still only 3 percent Black and 3.5 percent Hispanic physicians in the U.S. physician population.

The following are application, acceptance, and graduation rates for minority students taken from 1992 through 1997. In order to increase these numbers, many new programs have been initiated to help students become more competitive.

	1992	1993	1994	1995	1996	1997
African American						
Total Applicant Pool	2917	3489	3659	3595	3451	3133
Accepted Applicants	1291	1381	1427	1407	1244	1200
Native American						
Total Applicant Pool	194	238	261	305	374	311
Accepted Applicants	103	120	116	138	153	133
Mexican / Hispanic						
Total Applicant Pool	1964	2850	2895	3341	2830	2445
Accepted Applicants	1420	1389	1359	1409	1182	1043
Asian / Pacific Islander						
Total Applicant Pool	6225	7813	8804	9644	9065	8641
Accepted Applicants	2719	2754	2960	3122	3067	3311

As the trends indicate, there is a disturbing lack of minority applicants at the same time the minority population is increasing at a high rate. Even if current admission and graduation rates for minority students stabilize, the overall percentage of practicing minority physicians will actually drop compared to the total minority population. The good news is that this can be an exciting time for minority students to try and reverse that trend. Medical schools are aware of the potential shortage and are seeking good minority representation in their incoming classes. As a minority student interested in medicine, you're in an excellent position to gain admission if you're willing to do everything necessary to become the best qualified person you can be.

Preparing for Medical School

Although trends for minority students have changed, some of the problems these students face remain. If you're a minority student, and you've spent the last four years in a historically black college, the first hurdle you'll have to face is entering a predominantly white medical school. Like many other students, you may experience culture shock, defined as the anxiety resulting from a loss of familiar signs and symbols of social interaction. These signs or cues include the ways in which we orient ourselves to the situations of daily life. They may be words, speech patterns, gestures, facial expressions, and customs acquired by all of us in the course of growing up. They're often as much a part of our culture as the language we speak or the beliefs we accept, and are used in the interacting experience of day to day living with others in our own culture.

Another source of strain minority students often face is science preparation. Even though many minority students possess skills and scientific preparation equal to that of any other student, you may not because of reasons that were beyond your control. You need to prepare yourself to work harder on enhancing your science background and understanding. If you have problems with reading, then the amount of reading you'll have to do in medical school will overwhelm you. Remedial courses can improve study skills and are usually very helpful in developing better problem-solving and general academic skills. Since many students, including minority students, tend to rely on rote learning, courses designed to help build analytical thought processes and critical thinking are highly recommended. They'll also help you do better on the MCAT, which is a test designed to measure analytical ability.

One of the most important reasons to improve science preparedness is that, besides having undergraduate students with outstanding backgrounds, the applicant pool has recently been loaded with many graduate students and individuals from health fields who now want to go to medical school. As a result, medical schools have increased their admissions standards in the basic sciences, creating an even wider gap between the two groups of students. Minority students are now having to compete with an increasingly science educated applicant pool. In order to overcome any deficiencies you might have in your science background, or to help you get ready for a medical school curriculum, you should take advantage of any opportunity you can.

Medical Minority Application Registry (Med-MAR)

Your first opportunity to enhance your standing as a potential medical student is to register for the Medical Minority Applicant Registry when you take the MCAT. Med-MAR was started as a way to distribute biographical information of prospective minority students such as names, addresses, states of residence, racial/ethnic descriptions, undergraduate colleges, majors, and MCAT scores. To be eligible, you must meet two criteria:

1. You must be a U.S. citizen or permanent resident Visa holder
2. You must be African American, American Indian, Mexican American, or Mainland Puerto Rican

Medical schools use the registry (circulated twice a year following each MCAT) as a means of identifying and communicating with candidates. There is no cost to the student, so make sure you register when you take the exam.

Health Professions Partnership Initiative (HPPI)

The AAMC and the Robert Wood Johnson Foundation have initiated HPPI in order to increase the number of minority students prepared to go on to medical school. Grants are awarded to medical programs committed to increasing the diversity of the minority medical school applicant pool. The following medical schools have actively applied for and received grants to improve minority admissions. Their involvement in this program indicates a willingness on their part to help minority students enhance their chances for success. It would be a good idea to consider these medical programs when making your decision to apply to medical school.

Medical College of Georgia School of Medicine

Medical College of Pennsylvania and Hahnemann School of Medicine

Medical University of South Carolina College of Medicine

Oregon Health Sciences University School of Medicine

University of Connecticut School of Medicine

University of Louisville School of Medicine

University of Massachusetts Medical School

University of Nebraska College of Medicine

University of North Carolina at Chapel Hill School of Medicine

University of Wisconsin Medical School

Minority Medical Education Program (MMEP)

Students identified as underrepresented in the medical field by the Association of American Medical Colleges (AAMC) have an opportunity to participate in a 6-week summer enrichment program that help them compete for entrance into medical school. Some of the projects available through MMEP are: laboratory experiences with an M.D. or Ph.D. in clinical and research areas of medicine; academic classes in biology, math, and problem-solving; MCAT preparation; and counseling on medical school selection, application, and financing. To be eligible, a student must meet the following criteria:

1. Be a U.S. citizen or hold a permanent resident visa

2. Be African American, American Indian, Mexican American, mainland Puerto Rican, or Native Hawaiian

3. Have completed one year of college or have received a baccalaureate degree

4. Have an overall GPA of 3.0, with at least a 2.75 in science (individuals considered on case-by-case basis)

5. Have SAT or ACT scores of 950 or 20

6. Demonstrate a serious interest in medicine

Currently, there are nine medical schools participating in MMEP. They are listed below. You may contact them directly or get complete application materials and additional information from the MMEP National Program Office at:

Minority Medical Education Program
Association of American Medical Colleges
2450 N Street N.W.
Washington, D.C. 20037-1126
(202) 828-0401

University of Alabama School of Medicine
P-100 Volker Hall
Birmingham, AL 35294-0019
(800) 707-3579

Baylor College of Medicine
1709 Dryden, Suite 519
Houston, TX 77030
(713) 798-8200 or (800) 798-8244

University of Chicago Pritzker School of Medicine
924 E. 57th Street, BSLC104
Chicago, IL 60637-5416
(773) 702-1939

Fisk University and Vanderbilt University
1000 Seventeenth Avenue North
Nashville, TN 37208-3051
(615) 329-8796

University of Washington School of Medicine
SC-64
Seattle, WA 98195
(206) 685-2489

University of Arizona College of Medicine
1501 North Campbell Avenue, Room 1119-B
Tucson, AZ 85724
(602) 621-5531

Case Western Reserve University School of Medicine
10900 Euclid Avenue
Cleveland, OH 44106-4920
(216) 368-2212

University of Virginia School of Medicine
Box 446, HSC
Charlottesville, VA 22908
(804) 924-2189

Yale University School of Medicine
P.O. Box 208080
New Haven, CT 06520-8080
(203) 785-2129

Minority Summer Enrichment Programs

Summer enrichment programs not only help increase science knowledge and improve study skills, they force students to develop good study habits and teach them how to manage their time effectively. The principle behind many of these programs is to build academic endurance through the "mud on the wall theory." That is, get bombarded with enough information and something has to stick. Some programs are designed for students not yet accepted to medical school while others are strictly for students that have been accepted but need extra help in order to become more competitive.

A typical program consists of a very intense 8 to 5 academic workday, designed to simulate a first-year medical curriculum through lectures, movies, teaching aids, and seminars on subjects such as anatomy, physiology, biochemistry, etc. Some programs even include MCAT preparation sessions. A stipend is offered which varies from program to program. You may write to the individual programs for applications and detailed information about benefits offered such as room and board.

The instructors at these programs are often medical school faculty members, and some may even be admissions committee members. Therefore, doing well at these summer programs could make a difference in your getting admitted to a medical school.

ALABAMA

UNIVERSITY OF ALABAMA SCHOOL OF MEDICINE
Minority Medical Education Program (MMEP) P-100 Volker Hall
Birmingham, AL 35294-0019
(800) 707-3579
ELIGIBILITY: Underrepresented minority with at least one year of college or baccalaureate degree, an overall GPA of 3.0, and a science GPA of 2.75. Must have a demonstrated interest in a medical career.
PROGRAM LENGTH: 6 weeks
APPLICATION DEADLINE: April 1

ARIZONA

UNIVERSITY OF ARIZONA COLLEGE OF MEDICINE
Minority Medical Education Program (MMEP)
1501 North Campbell Avenue
Room 1119-B
Tucson, AZ 85724
(520) 621-5531
ELIGIBILITY: Underrepresented minority with at least one year of college or baccalaureate degree, an overall GPA of 3.0, and a science GPA of 2.75. Must have a demonstrated interest in a medical career.
PROGRAM LENGTH: 6 weeks
APPLICATION DEADLINE: April 1

CALIFORNIA

CHARLES R. DREW UNIVERSITY OF MEDICINE & SCIENCE
Summer MCAT Preparation Program
1621 E. 120th Street, MP#46A
Keck Building/Allied Health
Los Angeles, CA 90059
(213) 563-4926
ELIGIBILITY: Completion of medical school prerequisite courses and a minimum 2.1 science GPA.
PROGRAM LENGTH: 7 weeks
APPLICATION DEADLINE: March 31

SAN DIEGO STATE UNIVERSITY
Health Careers Opportunity Program
College of Sciences
LS 204
San Diego, CA 92182-0277
(619) 594-0277
ELIGIBILITY: Underrepresented minority SDSU student with overall GPA of 2.5 or better and a demonstrated interest in medicine.
PROGRAM LENGTH: 7 weeks
APPLICATION DEADLINE: March 15

SAN JOSE STATE UNIVERSITY
HCOP Summer Enrichment Program
College of Applied Sciences and Arts
One Washington Square
San Jose, CA 95192-0049
(408) 924-2911
ELIGIBILITY: Underrepresented minority or disadvantaged sophomore or junior student admitted to SJSU.
PROGRAM LENGTH: 6 weeks
APPLICATION DEADLINE: May 1

UNIVERSITY OF CALIFORNIA - IRVINE, COLLEGE OF MEDICINE
Summer Premedical Program
Office of Educational and Community Programs
UCI College of Medicine
P.O. Box 4089
Irvine, CA 92717
(714) 824-4603 or (800) 824-6442
ELIGIBILITY: Underrepresented minority or disadvantaged sophomore students pursuing a medical career.
PROGRAM LENGTH: 6 weeks
APPLICATION DEADLINE: March 15

UNIVERSITY OF CALIFORNIA LOS ANGELES SCHOOL OF MEDICINE
Summer Premedical Enrichment Program (UCLA PREP)
Office of Student Support Services
13-154 Center for the Health Sciences
Box 956990
Los Angeles, CA 90095-6990
(310) 825-3575
ELIGIBILITY: Disadvantaged students who have completed one year of college chemistry with a grade of C or better and an overall minimum GPA of 2.5
PROGRAM LENGTH: 8 weeks
APPLICATION DEADLINE: March 1

CONNECTICUT

UNIVERSITY OF CONNECTICUT HEALTH CENTER
Medical/Dental Preparatory Program (MDPP)
University of Connecticut Health Center
Office of Minority Student Affairs
Farmington, CT 06030-3920
(860) 679-3483
ELIGIBILITY: Underrepresented and highly motivated minority or disadvantaged sophomores, juniors, seniors, or recent graduates of pre-professional programs with a demonstrated interest in pursuing a degree in medicine or dentistry.
PROGRAM LENGTH: 6 weeks
APPLICATION DEADLINE: April 30

UNIVERSITY OF CONNECTICUT HEALTH CENTER
College Enrichment Program (CEP)
University of Connecticut Health Center
Office of Minority Student Affairs
Farmington, CT 06030-3920
(860) 679-3483

ELIGIBILITY: Underrepresented and highly motivated minority or disadvantaged freshman or sophomores with a demonstrated interest in a health career.

PROGRAM LENGTH: 6 weeks

APPLICATION DEADLINE: April 30

YALE UNIVERSITY SCHOOL OF MEDICINE

Minority Medical Education Program (MMEP)

P.O. Box 208080

New Haven, CT 06520-8080

(203) 785-2129

ELIGIBILITY: Underrepresented minorities who have completed at least one year of college or have a baccalaureate degree with an overall GPA of 3.0 and a science GPA of 2.75.

PROGRAM LENGTH: 6 weeks

APPLICATION DEADLINE: April 1

COLORADO

UNIVERSITY OF COLORADO HEALTH SCIENCE CENTER

Science Education and Enrichment Kaleidoscope (SEEK)

Center for Multicultural Enrichment

Box B-176, 4200 East 9th Avenue

Denver, CO 80262

(303) 270-8558

ELIGIBILITY: Underrepresented minorities who have completed at least two years of undergraduate science or pre-professional course work and plan to reapply for admission within the next two years.

PROGRAM LENGTH: 8 weeks

APPLICATION DEADLINE: March 30

DISTRICT OF COLUMBIA

HOWARD UNIVERSITY

Summer Health Careers Advanced Enrichment Program

Director, Center for Preprofessional Education

Box 473, Administration Building

Washington, DC 20059

(202) 806-7231

ELIGIBILITY: Disadvantaged juniors and seniors who have a minimum GPA of 2.5 and have completed the basic courses required by health professional schools.

PROGRAM LENGTH: 6 weeks

APPLICATION DEADLINE: April 30

FLORIDA

UNIVERSITY OF MIAMI SCHOOL OF MEDICINE

. Health Careers Motivation Program

P.O. Box 016960 (R 128)

Miami, FL 33101

(305) 243-5998

ELIGIBILITY: Underrepresented minority students who have completed two or three years of college with a focus on premedical studies.

PROGRAM LENGTH: 7 weeks

APPLICATION DEADLINE: April 30

GEORGIA

EMORY UNIVERSITY SCHOOL OF MEDICINE

Summer Minority MCAT Enrichment Program

Associate Dean, Office of Minority Affairs

WHSCAB, Room 314A

1440 Clifton Road, N.E.

Atlanta, GA 30322

(404) 727-0016

ELIGIBILITY: Underrepresented minority and disadvantaged students who have completed their junior year of college, have an overall GPA of 2.8, and are planning on taking the fall MCAT.

PROGRAM LENGTH: 6 weeks

APPLICATION DEADLINE: January 31

MEDICAL COLLEGE OF GEORGIA

Student Educational Enrichment Program in the Health Sciences

Suite AA-153

Augusta, GA 30912-1900

(706) 721-2522

ELIGIBILITY: Underrepresented minority and disadvantaged students in one of two groups: (A) Students who have finished their freshman or sophomore year with a 2.75 GPA, and (B) students who have finished the junior year with a GPA of 3.0.

PROGRAM LENGTH: 8 weeks

APPLICATION DEADLINE: March 1

ILLINOIS

RUSH MEDICAL COLLEGE

Chicago Summer Science Enrichment Program

Director, Minority Medical Education Program

1725 West Harrison Street

Chicago, IL 60612

(312) 942-5919

ELIGIBILITY: Underrepresented minority students who have completed at least one year of college and have an overall GPA of 3.0 and a science GPA of 2.75.

PROGRAM LENGTH: 6 weeks

APPLICATION DEADLINE: April 1

ILLINOIS INSTITUTE OF TECHNOLOGY
Chicago Area Health and Medical Careers Program (CAHMCP)
Commons Building
3200 S. Wabash Avenue
Chicago, IL 60616-3793
(312) 567-3890
ELIGIBILITY: Underrepresented minority students who have completed at least one year of college and have an overall GPA of 3.0 and a science GPA of 2.75. SAT/ACT scores should be 950/15. Preference is given to Illinois residents.
PROGRAM LENGTH: 7 weeks
APPLICATION DEADLINE: April 1

UNIVERSITY OF ILLINOIS COLLEGE OF MEDICINE
Summer Academic Enrichment Program
Urban Health Program / Hispanic Center of Excellence
1819 West Polk Street
Room 145 CMW (m/c 786)
Chicago, IL 60612
(312) 996-6491
ELIGIBILITY: Underrepresented minority or disadvantaged students who have completed the sophomore year of college and successfully completed science courses in biology and chemistry. Must be an Illinois resident.
PROGRAM LENGTH: 8 weeks
APPLICATION DEADLINE: April 30

LOUISIANA

TULANE UNIVERSITY SCHOOL OF MEDICINE
Medical Education Reinforcement and Enrichment Program (MEdREP)
Associate Dean for Student Services
Director of MEdREP
1430 Tulane Avenue - SL40
New Orleans, LA 70112-2699
ELIGIBILITY: Minority or disadvantaged students who have completed at least two years of college or premedical training.
PROGRAM LENGTH: 8 weeks
APPLICATION DEADLINE: March 1

MARYLAND

ADVANCED PREMEDICAL DEVELOPMENT PROGRAM (APDP)
Program Administrator
Office of Student and Faculty Development
655 West Baltimore Street, M-004
Baltimore, MD 21201
ELIGIBILITY: Minority or disadvantaged rising seniors or recent college graduates with a GPA of 3.3 or better and completion of prerequisite biology, chemistry, and physics.

PROGRAM LENGTH: 6 weeks
APPLICATION DEADLINE: March 15

MASSACHUSETTS

UNIVERSITY OF MASSACHUSETTS MEDICAL CENTER
Summer Enrichment Program (SEP)
Office of Outreach Programs
UMASS Medical Center
55 Lake Avenue North, S1-844
Worcester, MA 01655-0132
(508) 856-5541
ELIGIBILITY: Underrepresented minority or economically disadvantaged students who are residents of Massachusetts, or will be when they enter medical school, and have completed 8 hours of organic chemistry and 30 hours of college course work.
PROGRAM LENGTH: 4 weeks
APPLICATION DEADLINE: March 1

MINNESOTA

MAYO SCHOOL OF HEALTH-RELATED SCIENCES
Mayo Medical School
Director, Summer Enrichment Program
Rochester, MN 55905
ELIGIBILITY: Rising juniors or seniors
PROGRAM LENGTH: Contact Mayo
APPLICATION DEADLINE: February 16

NEW YORK

ALBERT EINSTEIN COLLEGE OF MEDICINE
Sue Golding Graduate Division of Medical Sciences
1300 Morris Park Avenue
Bronx, NY 10461
ELIGIBILITY: Undergraduate students who are juniors and have a strong interest in a Ph.D. or M.D./Ph.D.
PROGRAM LENGTH: 10 weeks
APPLICATION DEADLINE: March 1

CORNELL UNIVERSITY MEDICAL COLLEGE
Travelers Summer Research Fellowship Program for Premedical Minority Students
445 East 69th Street, Room 110
New York, NY 10021
(212) 746-1057
ELIGIBILITY: Minority premedical students who have completed their junior year of college.
PROGRAM LENGTH: 7 weeks
APPLICATION DEADLINE: March 1

NEW YORK UNIVERSITY SCHOOL OF MEDICINE

Minority Undergraduate Research Program (S.U.R.P.)

Sackler Institute

550 First Avenue

New York, NY 10016

(212) 263-5649

ELIGIBILITY: Students who have completed their junior year of college and plan to pursue a career as an M.D./Ph.D.

PROGRAM LENGTH: 8 weeks

APPLICATION DEADLINE: February 1

NORTH CAROLINA

WAKE FOREST UNIVERSITY SCHOOL OF MEDICINE

Health Careers Opportunity Program

Office of Minority Affairs

Medical Center Boulevard

Winston-Salem, NC 27157-1037

(919) 748-4201

ELIGIBILITY: Underrepresented minority college freshman or sophomores with a minimum GPA of 2.5 and a demonstrated potential for a career in medicine.

PROGRAM LENGTH: 6 weeks

APPLICATION DEADLINE: April 1

EAST CAROLINA UNIVERSITY SCHOOL OF MEDICINE

Summer Program for Future Doctors

2N45 Brody Medical Sciences Building

Greenville, NC 27858-4354

(919) 816-2500

ELIGIBILITY: Underrepresented minority, disadvantaged, and non-traditional students who have completed introductory level biology, chemistry, and physics. Preference is given to North Carolina residents.

PROGRAM LENGTH: 8 weeks

APPLICATION DEADLINE: March 1

UNIVERSITY OF NORTH CAROLINA at CHAPEL HILL

Summer Enrichment Preparation Program

CB# 8010, 301 Pittsboro Street, Suite 351

Chapel Hill, NC 27599-8010

(919) 966-2264

ELIGIBILITY: Underrepresented minority, disadvantaged, and non-traditional students who have completed their sophomore or junior year and have a minimum GPA of 2.5. Preference is given to North Carolina residents.

PROGRAM LENGTH: 8 weeks

APPLICATION DEADLINE: March 1

NORTH DAKOTA

UNIVERSITY OF NORTH DAKOTA
Indians into Medicine Program (INMED)
INMED Program
501 North Columbia Road
Grand Forks, ND 58203
(701) 777-3037
ELIGIBILITY: Ten Native American students
PROGRAM LENGTH: 6 weeks
APPLICATION DEADLINE: March 31

OHIO

CASE WESTERN RESERVE UNIVERSITY SCHOOL OF MEDICINE
Health Careers Enhancement Program for Minorities (HCEM)
10900 Euclid Avenue
Cleveland, OH 44106-4920
(216) 368-2212
ELIGIBILITY: Underrepresented minority students with an overall GPA of 3.0, a science GPA of 2.75, and combined SAT/ACT scores of 950/20.
PROGRAM LENGTH: 6 weeks
APPLICATION DEADLINE: April 1

THE METROHEALTH FOUNDATION
Edward M. Chester, M.D. Summer Scholars Program
2500 Metro Health Drive
Cleveland, OH 44109-1998
(216) 778-5665
ELIGIBILITY: Students who have completed two undergraduate years in premedical or scientific study. Must be a resident of Ohio or attend an Ohio college or university
PROGRAM LENGTH: 8 weeks
APPLICATION DEADLINE: January 15

OHIO STATE UNIVERSITY COLLEGE OF MEDICINE
MEDPATH Program
1072 Graves Hall
Columbus, OH 43210
(614) 292-3161
ELIGIBILITY: Underrepresented minority or disadvantaged nonscience majors who have already been accepted into a medical school and who need additional preparation prior to entrance.
PROGRAM LENGTH: 6 weeks
APPLICATION DEADLINE: Contact program

UNIVERSITY OF CINCINNATI COLLEGE OF MEDICINE
Summer Premedical Enrichment Program (SPEP)
231 Bethesda Avenue
Cincinnati, OH 45267-0552
(513) 558-7212
ELIGIBILITY: Underrepresented minority or disadvantaged students who have completed two years of undergraduate work.
PROGRAM LENGTH: 8 weeks
APPLICATION DEADLINE: March 1

OKLAHOMA

UNIVERSITY OF OKLAHOMA HEALTH SCIENCES CENTER
Headlands Indian Health Careers Summer Academic Enrichment Program
Headlands Indian Health Careers
BSEB - Room 200
P.O. Box 26901
Oklahoma City, OK 73126-9968
(405) 271-2250
ELIGIBILITY: American Indian students in their senior year of high school or first year of college who have completed at least two years of algebra, two science courses, and have a 2.5 GPA.
PROGRAM LENGTH: 8 weeks
APPLICATION DEADLINE: March 15

SOUTH CAROLINA

MEDICAL UNIVERSITY OF SOUTH CAROLINA
Summer Health Careers Opportunity Program (HCOP)
Office of Diversity
171 Ashley Avenue
Charleston, SC 29425-1018
(803) 792-8484
ELIGIBILITY: Juniors who have completed one year of biology and chemistry through organic chemistry and have a GPA of 2.5 or better in math and science.
PROGRAM LENGTH: 8 weeks
APPLICATION DEADLINE: April 25

TENNESSEE

EAST TENNESSEE STATE UNIVERSITY COLLEGE OF MEDICINE
Preprofessional Reinforcement and Enrichment Program (PREP)
PREP Coordinator
Office of Student Affairs
P.O. Box 70580
Johnson City, TN 37614-0580
(423) 439-5655

ELIGIBILITY: Underrepresented minority and disadvantaged students currently enrolled in a post-secondary institution and who have completed one year of college biology and chemistry. Preference given to Tennessee residents.
PROGRAM LENGTH: 8 weeks
APPLICATION DEADLINE: Contact program

FISK UNIVERSITY/VANDERBILT UNIVERSITY
United Negro College Fund
Premedical Summer Institute
Fisk University
1000 Seventeenth Avenue North
Nashville, TN 37208-3051
(615) 329-8796
ELIGIBILITY: Underrepresented minority and disadvantaged students with an overall GPA of 3.0, a science GPA of 2.75, combined SAT or ACT scores of 950 or 20, and a serious interest in a medical career.
PROGRAM LENGTH: 6 weeks
APPLICATION DEADLINE: April 1

MEHARRY MEDICAL COLLEGE
Biomedical Science Program (BSP)
1005 D.B. Todd Boulevard
Nashville, TN 37208
(615) 327-6533
ELIGIBILITY: Underrepresented minority students who have completed their freshman or sophomore year with an overall B average and a B average in science and math
PROGRAM LENGTH: 8 weeks
APPLICATION DEADLINE: March 25

TEXAS

BAYLOR COLLEGE OF MEDICINE/RICE UNIVERSITY
Honors Premedical Academy (HPA)
Minority Medical Education Program (MMEP)
1709 Dryden, Suite 545
Houston, TX 77030
(713) 798-8200
ELIGIBILITY: Underrepresented minority students who have completed their first year of college, have an overall GPA of 3.0, a science GPA of 2.75, and combined SAT or ACT scores of at least 950 or 20. Students must have a demonstrated serious interest in a medical career.
PROGRAM LENGTH: 6 weeks
APPLICATION DEADLINE: April 1

TEXAS A&M UNIVERSITY COLLEGE OF MEDICINE
Bridge to Medicine MCAT Program (BTM)
Program Director

106 Joe H. Reynolds Medical Building

College Station, TX 77843-1114

(409) 862-4065

ELIGIBILITY: Disadvantaged students who have completed at least four semesters of undergraduate coursework and have a good overall GPA.

PROGRAM LENGTH: 6 weeks

APPLICATION DEADLINE: March 1

UNIVERSITY OF TEXAS HEALTH SCIENCE CENTER at SAN ANTONIO

MCAT Performance Improvement Program

Program Director

Pyramid Plaza

7434 Louis Pasteur, Suite 209

San Antonio, TX 78229

(210) 614-1435

ELIGIBILITY: All college students who have completed at least four semesters of undergraduate coursework (60 hours) and have a good overall GPA. The program focuses mainly on juniors, seniors, or postgraduate students.

PROGRAM LENGTH: 6 weeks

APPLICATION DEADLINE: March 1

VIRGINIA

VIRGINIA COMMONWEALTH UNIVERSITY MEDICAL COLLEGE OF VIRGINIA

MCV Health Careers Opportunity Program

P.O. Box 980549

Richmond, VA 23298-0549

(804) 828-4200

ELIGIBILITY: Minority students currently enrolled in a college or university or who have graduated and have demonstrated a desire to pursue a medical career.

PROGRAM LENGTH: 6 weeks

APPLICATION DEADLINE: April 4

UNIVERSITY OF VIRGINIA SCHOOL OF MEDICINE

Medical Academic Advancement Programs (MAAP)

Minority Medical Education Programs (MMEP)

Box 446, HSC

Charlottesville, VA

(804) 243-6165

ELIGIBILITY: Minority sophomores, juniors, seniors, or current graduates who have an overall GPA of 3.0, a science GPA of 2.75, a combined SAT or ACT score of 950 or 20, and a serious interest in pursuing a career in medicine.

PROGRAM LENGTH: 6 weeks

APPLICATION DEADLINE: May 1

WASHINGTON

UNIVERSITY OF WASHINGTON SCHOOL OF MEDICINE
Minority Medical Education Program (MMEP)
Program Director
Box 357430
Seattle, WA 98195
(206) 685-2489
ELIGIBILITY: Underrepresented minority students who have completed at least one year of college or who have graduated, have an overall GPA of 3.0, a science GPA of 2.75, and have a demonstrated serious interest in a medical career.
PROGRAM LENGTH: 6 weeks
APPLICATION DEADLINE: April 1

Some Final Suggestions for Minority Students

Currently, minority applicants have an overall acceptance rate of 40 percent compared to a 50 percent acceptance rate five years earlier. This is occurring even though minority applicants are far better qualified now than they were a decade or so ago and have their mean MCAT scores closer to those of their majority counter-parts. The problem lies not in qualifications but in the social hurdles many minority students still have to over-come on the way to a career in medicine. According to the former dean of student affairs at Stanford University School of Medicine, "Things will only get worse before they get better."

Because of financial impacts, increasing numbers of minorities below the poverty line face a much tougher road on their way to medical school. Minority youngsters are more likely to attend elementary and high schools in high poverty areas characterized by low academic performance, discipline problems, low levels of parental involvement, and less qualified and unmotivated teachers. The cumulative impact of these factors begins to show up in lower educational achievement by about age ten. Minority students are often placed into vocational courses or in low-track classes where they are not intellectually challenged, where expectations are low and where the message is sent that they cannot aspire to higher scholastic achievement. Add to this rising tuition rates, low graduation rates from high school, lack of role models, and increasing interest in other professions such as business, and you have an alarming trend of very few minorities pursuing medicine as a career.

The good news is that, because minority medical admissions have leveled off or are declining, more attention than ever is being paid to the characteristics of the minority applicant pool, it's qualifications, and size. Medical schools and premedical programs are serious about reversing the trend and are focusing on ways to improve academic skills and MCAT scores, providing role models and mentors, and providing financial assistance. Today, achieving greater minority representation in medical school and other health professions depends increasingly on improving a student's overall performance and his or her ability to compete in an educational environment that places a premium on credentials and quantitative skills. Besides the areas already mentioned, here are some suggestions for improving your chances of being a successful medical school applicant.

1. Minority students who participate in high school or college science and math enrichment programs are more likely to be accepted into medical school than non-participants. College-level enrichment programs that have proven particularly valuable in improving medical school acceptance rates are educational programs that provide a summer laboratory experience. You need to take advantage of any opportunity that will enhance your academic credentials.

2. Too few minority high school and college students take advanced science and math courses. Math and science skills directly affect performance on standardized tests and are gatekeepers to higher education. Programs that include MCAT preparation, for example, can improve test scores significantly. This alone could mean the difference between acceptance and rejection.

One of the biggest trouble spots minority students have is the MCAT. Preparation courses are beneficial because they actually teach you how to take the MCAT exam.

3. Unless a student gets really serious from day one, college may be too late to improve academic skills and knowledge of science and math. Therefore, preparation should really begin in high school. According to statistics, a student's MCAT performance could be predicted accurately from scores on the SAT taken in the last year of high school. This finding suggests that, to maximize your chances for success, you need to take high school seriously.

4. Minority students who apply to five or more medical schools and who receive help with the application process are more likely to be accepted than those who don't. Applying to more schools will increase the chances that your qualifications, credentials, and background will match the admissions criteria of a given school.

5. Non-academic factors such as poor guidance counseling and insufficient career information contribute greatly to the loss of minorities from the medical applicant pool. If your school doesn't have a good guidance counselor or lacks information, don't be afraid to go somewhere else for advice. Also, never assume that your counselor knows what's best for you or even that he or she has your best interests at heart. Dr. Benjamin Carson, the world famous black neurosurgeon who performed one of the first operations to separate Siamese twins joined at the head, was told by his advisor that he was not smart enough to be a doctor. Dr. Carson was smart enough to ignore that advice!

6. Having minority physicians as role models and mentors is key to many minority students' success. Role models and mentors provide valuable standards of achievement, inspire career choices, and lay out avenues for upward mobility. You need to find a role model or mentor from medical school, from your community, or your hospital. These role models will help you compensate for the isolation you'll often encounter in academic and professional settings where you'll no doubt be underrepresented. More than anything else, your mentor will encourage you when things get tough, and give you the needed inspiration you need to keep going.

Recently, I had the privilege of meeting Dr. Benjamin Carson who, at the age of 38, was already chief of pediatric surgery at Johns Hopkins University School of Medicine. He'd spoken at NC A&T State University to students interested in health careers. The message he brought was simple: "Anyone can do anything they want if they set their mind to it and are prepared to work hard to achieve their goals." He went on to say that "Blacks and other minorities have every opportunity to pursue health careers and can rise as far as they are willing to go."

From a Detroit ghetto, where he almost destroyed his life, to Yale University, and finally to medical school, Dr. Carson became one of only a handful of black neurosurgeons in the world. The reason: He never stopped believing that he was capable of doing whatever he set out to do. You, too, can follow that example and achieve your goal of medical school if you're willing to work hard for it. With enough desire and determination, your chances of gaining admission to medical school are much better than you think.

10

Foreign Medical Education

One of the last options you may want to consider if you're unsuccessful in gaining admission to medical school is to apply to one or more foreign medical schools. There's no accurate way to determine just how many students choose the option of studying abroad, but it's believed that the numbers have been steadily increasing because of the record number of applicants vying for limited space in U.S. medical programs.

There are excellent medical schools throughout the world, especially in Europe. There are also a few that offer their curriculums entirely in English (the Philippines and the Caribbean, for example). Many foreign medical schools, however, will not accept applications from the United States and, therefore, you need to plan carefully. For instance, some of the countries currently not accepting applications from U.S. citizens are Australia, Austria, Ireland, Italy, Great Britain, south Africa, and Switzerland. Canadian medical schools are not considered "foreign" by the AAMC, but accept only a very few American students each year.

Before you decide on applying to any foreign medical school, I want to urge you to consider seriously other options. The government accounting office (GAO) has visited many foreign schools which account for nearly half of all enrolled U.S. citizens and found that they differ considerably. In the GAO's opinion, none of the foreign medical schools offered a medical education comparable to that available in the United States due to serious deficiencies in admission requirements, equipment, faculty, curriculum, and clinical training. Although it's difficult to judge foreign schools in all these areas, a serious shortcoming at each school was the lack of adequate clinical training facilities.

World's Most Prestigious Foreign Medical Schools

None of the foreign medical schools examined by the government accounting office had access to the same range of clinical facilities and numbers and variety of patients as United States programs. Many of these schools are located in poor countries that lack modern conveniences. Caribbean schools have been especially suspect in recent years because of serious curriculum deficiencies and poor teaching facilities.

The following table lists some of the most prestigious foreign medical schools throughout the world, based on facilities, teaching faculty, and the rigors of medical training the students get. The schools are listed in alphabetical order.

Brussels University, Belgium

Cambridge University, United Kingdom

Dijon University, France

Edinburgh University, United Kingdom (Scotland)

Geneva University, Switzerland

Gottingen University, Germany

Heidelberg University, Germany

Lille (Faculte Libre de Medicine), France

Lille (U.E.R.) University, France

Lyon 1 University, France

McGill University, Canada

Montpellier University, France

Munich University, Germany

Oxford University, United Kingdom

Toronto University, Canada

Vienna University, Austria

Zurich University, Switzerland

Medical Education in Europe

Many students choose to apply to European medical schools rather than other foreign schools because of Europe's good track record in offering a good medical education. In the past, many European medical schools required only a secondary school diploma, but during the last few decades a more formal and stringent selection process has become necessary due, naturally, to the increasing complexity of medicine and the increasing numbers of both national and international applicants. Here are some interesting facts about a few select medical schools in Europe and what they use to select their medical students. The list is by no means complete, but it should give you an idea of what you'd be up against when considering this path.

1. All countries, with the exception of Belgium, Italy, and Switzerland, have special citizenry requirements for entrance to medical school.

2. In almost every country, the average age of candidates at the time of selection is 20 in contrast to the United States medical school average age of 25. There's more of a tendency for European medial schools to take age into consideration than it is for medical schools in the United States.

3. In general, there's a growing tendency to admit more women applicants. The current rate is somewhere between 25 and 30 percent, compared to more than 40 percent in the United States.

4. Different countries often have very different entrance requirements. For example, in Germany, 60 percent of admissions is based on scores of undergraduate exams. In the Netherlands, entrance is based on overall science scores on the final secondary school examinations. In Sweden, grades obtained during the final years of secondary school are taken into consideration.

5. Because of limited space and facilities, some countries such as Germany and the Netherlands have lottery systems for admitting students who were not accepted immediately.

6. Some countries such as the Netherlands, Denmark, and Sweden make special allowances for students who have served in the armed forces or who have participated in a medically-related activity or job.

Educational Commission for Foreign Medical Graduates (ECFMG)

Through its program of certification, the ECFMG ensures that graduates of foreign medical schools are, indeed, competent to practice medicine in the United States. It defines a foreign medical school graduate as any physician, regardless of nationality, who has received training and a degree from a medical school located outside the United States, Canada, and Puerto Rico, and which is listed in the *World Directory of Medical Schools* published by the World Health Organization.

ECFMG certification is required for licensure to practice medicine in the United States. Furthermore, it assesses the readiness of graduates to enter residency or fellowship programs; and, therefore, without ECFMG certification, a graduate of a foreign medical school cannot become a resident. The following are requirements for ECFMG certification effective July 1, 1998:

1. **Pass the basic medical and clinical science components of the medical science examination within a seven year period**. This is basically step 1 (basic medical) and step 2 (clinical) of the United States Medical Licensing Examination (USMLE) typically administered by the Federation of State Medical Boards (FSMB) and National Board of Medical Examiners (NBME).

2. **Pass the English language proficiency test**. Passing performance on the English test is valid for two years from the date passed for purposes of entry into graduate medical education.

3. **Pass the Clinical Skills Assessment (CSA), including an assessment of spoken English proficiency**. This is a one-day exam that requires a demonstration of both clinical proficiency *and* spoken English language proficiency. Applicants must

pass the basic medical and clinical science component and the English proficiency test as prerequisites for the CSA. There is no limit on the amount of time which may elapse between these prerequisite examinations and CSA. Passing performance on CSA is valid for three years from the date passed for purposes of entry into graduate medical education.

4. **Document the completion of all requirements for, and receipt of, the final medical diploma.** All graduates of foreign medical schools must have at least four years (academic years for which credit has been given toward completion of the medical curriculum) in attendance at a medical school listed in the World Directory of Medical Schools at the time of graduation. In the event that a medical school is not listed in the directory, the ECFMG will consider applications on a case-by-case basis.

For more information on foreign medical school education you may write for information from:

ECFMG
3624 Market Street
4th Floor
Philadelphia, PA 19104-2685
(215) 386-5900

Choosing the Best Foreign Medical School

If you haven't been accepted to any United States medical school, I would strongly recommend that you try several more times before opting for the foreign school route. Even though there were almost 50,000 applicants vying for U.S. medical schools last year, there were approximately 16,000 openings, an acceptance rate of 32 percent. That means one-third of all applicants get in somewhere, which is much better odds than many foreign medical schools would give you.

Chances are, if you plan a little better, improve your academic standing, and increase your participation in extracurricular activities, you'll become one of the successful candidates the second or even third time around. One of the best ways to improve those chances, if your academic credentials are not great, is to establish residence in a state with several medical schools. The more medical schools, the better the odds. By becoming a resident, gaining a year's work experience, and enhancing your social and civic activities, you should be able to get into one of the state medical colleges.

If all else fails, and you've tried repeatedly to gain admission, you must still look very carefully and intelligently at your choices of foreign schools. The drop-out rate for non-foreign students at these colleges is quite high. Almost 70 percent of first year medical students leave before or after completed their freshman year. And a high percentage of those who *do* make it through four years can't transfer back into the United States for residency programs.

The reasons for the high failure rates vary, but they have a lot to do with how the students themselves choose the school. Most students simply don't get enough information about the school to make a good judgment. Consequently, they waste their time and money on a poor medical education that won't even allow them to come back to the states. You can't imagine the number of bad medical schools that prey on desperate premedical students who'll pay any price to get admitted and become doctors. These programs count on that. Unfortunately, the probability that these students will receive a first-rate medical education is fairly low. Here are some questions you may want to ask yourself before deciding to apply to any foreign medical school:

1. What language is the curriculum taught in? Are you particularly strong in that language and, if not, will you be by the time you enter? If you think medical school is tough, you haven't seen anything till you try it in another language.

2. Are the clinical facilities comparable to those in the United States or other international schools with good reputations? Much of a medical education is not classroom time but clinical time. Unless a medical school can offer you quality exposure, you're not going to get the proper training required to be successful in the United States.

3. Is the coursework and the course load similar to that offered by medical schools in the United States? Compare brochures and catalogues and see for yourself if the foreign school is shortchanging you. If the curriculum seems too easy, or if the coursework doesn't involve a wide variety of subject matter, it's not a good sign that the program is rigorous enough.

4. What's the graduation and failure rate of United States students who have gone to a particular foreign medical school? This will give you a good indication of what to expect. To get the latest results of how U.S. citizens have done on the ECFMG examination, write directly to ECFMG and request the statistics.

Deciding which foreign medical school is best for you will be especially important when you finally try to reenter the United States to practice medicine or to apply to a residency program. In recent years, less than 40 percent of U.S. citizens passed the ECFMG examination, which indicates that many foreign medical schools are not doing a good job preparing students for medical practice.

To give you an idea of how foreign medical school have stacked up against each other in years past in terms of success rate of the ECFMG exam, I've included the following list of countries and their pass rates. When making comparisons, though, you should be careful, since applicants for ECFMG examinations are self-selected, the data do not take into account the age of the examinees, the length of time between completion of training and the exam, the number of times the exam was taken, and other factors that may have affected the results. The point, however, is that students, on average and overall, did not fare very well when they graduated from foreign medical schools.

Country	Number Examined	Number Passed	Percent Passed
Belgium	27	20	74
Columbia	279	3	3
Dominican Republic	2692	577	21
France	36	25	69
Germany	47	29	62
Greece	63	17	27
Grenada	192	160	83
Guatemala	17	8	47
India	23	14	61
Ireland	21	16	76
Israel	51	51	100
Italy	352	135	38
Korea	26	14	54
Mexico	2132	738	35
Montserrat	360	186	52
Philippines	235	102	43
Poland	75	36	48
Romania	38	12	32
Spain	335	62	19

Returning to the United States

The ultimate goal of any medical student studying abroad is to return to the United States as a third year student or to enter into a U.S. residency program. Unfortunately, the number of residency openings throughout the United States is beginning to equal the number of yearly U.S. medical school graduates. Moreover, with the health care system making every effort to reduce costs, there may be less opportunity for certain residencies in the future. When it comes right down to it, foreign medical school graduates, unless they've studied at one of the top notch institutions, and even if they had, will always get last preference.

According to one survey, over 60 percent of foreign medical school graduates were not placed in residency programs. Some of these graduates had to do volunteer work in their selected residency specialty. To make matters worse, the number of American graduates of foreign medical schools applying for United States residencies has more than tripled recently, reducing even further the chances of getting into a residency program or even being able to volunteer altogether. The number of third year places in U.S. medical schools isn't expected to change either and, so, it's also unlikely that your chances of transferring into a medical school during your third or fourth year would be any better. Bottom line: graduating from a foreign medical school is not the way to go if you want to be at all competitive with U.S. graduates.

In general, there are three main ways by which foreign medical students can return to the United States to continue their medical education or to practice medicine. These are: (1) Transfer, (2) Certification, and (3) Fifth Pathway. Let's looks at each pathway individually.

1. *Transfer:* As mentioned, there are only a few places available in U. S. medical schools for transfer students from foreign medical schools. In order to obtain advanced placement, students need to take Part I of the USMLE administered by the National Board of Medical Examiners. In the past, fewer than 15 percent of all students taking the exam scored higher than the 50th percentile. And during the last few years, the actual number of U.S. citizens admitted as transfer students with advanced standing has declined more than 30 percent. Even passing the exam doesn't necessarily mean automatic admission to a U.S. medical school.

2. *Certification:* Students who have already graduated from a foreign medical school must take a special examination given by the Educational Commission for Foreign Medical School Graduates (ECFMG) twice a year, in January and July. Any foreign medical graduate who possesses an ECFMG certificate may participate in residency programs throughout the United States, though it doesn't guarantee that a place will be available. ECFMG recognizes only those foreign medical school graduates who have completed their medical training at institutions listed in the World Directory of Medical Schools. In the past, only about 16 percent of U.S. citizen graduates of foreign medical schools have passed the board's certifying examination compared with more than 80 percent of U.S. medical school graduates.

3. *Fifth Pathway:* By this avenue, foreign medical school graduates may apply for a year of clinical training in the United States after passing the ECFMG examination. The clinical training is the same as the clinical clerkships discussed in an earlier chapter. Like the other pathways, however, this one is also difficult, especially since there are very few positions available. Information on returning to the United States and practicing medicine may be obtained by writing to:

American Medical Association
515 North State Street
Chicago, IL 60610

Students who plan on applying to a foreign medical school need to know what they're getting them-selves into. They should get as much information from the foreign medical school as possible, they need to contact ECFMG for guidelines on testing, and they should contact the AMA with any questions they have on practicing medicine in the United States.

11

Financing A Medical Education

Money can certainly create a lot of problems if you're interested in getting a good medical education and are afraid of what it will cost you. The lack of money, however, doesn't have to keep you from considering a medical career. Many sources of financial aid are available, some geared specifically toward helping minority or disadvantaged students. But anyone can find sources of financial aid - scholarships, loans, work-study - if he or she is willing to look for them.

No medical school will turn an applicant away because of finances. Many students from poor backgrounds have been very successful in medical school, despite the difficulty they faced financially. Like thousands of others, you, too, can get through medical school regardless of your financial position and family background. The best way to ensure that you know about all the possibilities regarding financial aid is to consult the financial aid officer and student services director at the school and to shop around as early as possible for summer job opportunities.

Employment and Financial Aid

Because of the academic demands placed on medical students, most medical schools discourage employment, full or part-time, during the school year, especially during the first two years of the curriculum. Not all schools frown on part-time work, however; and there are a few that will even assist medical students in finding suitable work, so long as they keep their grades up. Having been affiliated with a medical school, and seeing what medical students go through, I would definitely recommend that a medical student find some sort of financial aid and not even attempt to work.

If accepted to medical school, it will be up to you to find out about financial aid from the school's financial aid department. Contact the financial aid officer soon after you've been notified of your acceptance and request that financial aid applications be sent to you. Normally, financial assistance is based on financial need, but a limited number of schools also offer scholarships, grants, and awards based on demonstrated academic excellence. When you receive the applications, complete them as soon as you can and send them in to be processed.

Other sources of financial aid besides the various awards offered by medical schools are available to qualified applicants. The sooner you apply and get an award, the sooner you can stop worrying about money and start concentrating on doing well your first year of medical school. Counseling is readily available at all medical schools, and the qualified staff will ensure that you'll get some sort of assistance during your four years.

MEDLOAN

Sponsored by the Association of American Medical Colleges (AAMC) in affiliation with leading financial U.S. financial institutions, MEDLOANS are one of the principle ways that students are able to support themselves during medical school. The program includes various borrowing options such as government or private loan guarantees, and a loan called MEDEX, which assists students who are beginning their residency programs.

MEDLOANS feature competitive interest rates and an array of incentives to help reduce payments. To find out more about the program call 1-800-858-5050.

Need-Based Financial Aid

Many schools place a high priority on need-based financial assistance for it's student's in the form of grants, low-interest loans, or a combination of both. At one particular school, for example, more than 80 percent of the total student enrollment received financial assistance from a source other than parents. Some schools would rather offer grants to needy students than loans in order to minimize the student's loan debt following graduation.

Need-based financial aid is offered to both state resident and non-resident students and it can vary from school to school. Typically, a medical school will also have a number of endowed scholarships, and students are selected for these based on specific criteria established by the donor of the scholarship. Because a student is usually considered for these at the same time he or she is being considered for all other types of financial aid, a separate application is not necessary. You should check the individual school, however, for any specific rules or deadlines, etc.

Merit Awards

Merit awards are based on academic excellence, and may have certain criteria attached to them such as minority status, extracurricular activities, or service and/or leadership in the community. Each medical school has a limited number of these merit scholarships, but they can be substantial. Full tuition for four years, as an example. Annual renewal of awards is often contingent upon satisfactory academic progress, which is defined by the medical school. In some cases, merit awards are only given to residents of the state in which the medical school is located. Others are open to any applicant. You need to check with the financial aid officer to see if you qualify.

Federal Government Assistance Programs

Many of the loans and grants available to medical students are offered through federal government agencies. As soon as you're accepted to a medical school, you should fill out a Free Application for Federal Student Aid (FAFSA) form. These are described below:

ARMED FORCES SCHOLARSHIP PROGRAM

These graduate scholarships are open to accepted students of medicine and other health-related careers such as dentistry, optometry, podiatry, etc. In return for a scholarship that covers all basic educational expenses such as tuition, fees, books and supplies and includes a monthly stipend, students must agree to serve one year in the military for each year of support. Further information is available by calling any recruiter of the Army, Navy, or Air Force or by writing to:

Office of the Assistant Secretary of Defense for Health Affairs

Room 3D, Pentagon

Washington, DC 20301

FEDERAL STAFFORD LOAN

Formerly known as the Guaranteed Student Loan or GSL, the Federal Stafford Loan is based on financial need and is the most common type of financial assistance for medical students. Two types of loan programs are available:

Subsidized Federal Stafford Loan: Students may borrow an annual maximum amount of $8,500 and a four-year total of $65,500. Interests rates vary from year to year and are based on a 91-day Treasury Bill plus 3.1% capped at 9%.

Unsubsidized Federal Stafford Loan: Students may receive unsubsidized funding up to $30,000 in addition to the $8,500 subsidized amount and a four year total of $138,500. Here, the student - not the federal government - is responsible for payment of the interest during enrollment and deferment periods.

The terms of each loan are different. Funds are distributed to the school via electronic mail and made payable to both the student and the institution. To be eligible, a medical student must meet one of the following criteria in order to be considered financially independent of parents:

1. Be at least 24 years old by December 31 of the award year.

2. Be an orphan or ward of the court.

3. Be a veteran of the Armed Forces of the United States.

4. Have legal dependents other than a spouse.

5. Be a graduate or professional student.

6. Be a married person who will not be claimed as an income tax exemption.

7. Be a single person with no dependents who was not claimed as a dependent by his or her parents.

FINANCIAL AID FOR DISADVANTAGED HEALTH PROFESSIONS STUDENTS (FADHPS)

Applicants for FADHPS are selected by the medical school based on financial need and federal guidelines. The main criteria is that the student be from a disadvantaged background or from a low income family. The student's financial resources must not exceed the lesser of $5,000 or one half of the cost of the medical education.

Following graduation, the student must enter a residency program in the primary health care field not later than four years after completing his or her medical education, then practice in primary care for five years after completion of the residency. Students who fail to meet academic standards or graduates who fail to comply with the primary care requirements will be liable to the federal government for the amount of the award plus any interest.

HEALTH EDUCATION ASSISTANCE LOAN (HEAL)

The HEAL program is a "need-based" federal loan program from the Department of Health and Human Services (DHHS) and is used as a supplemental resource after exhausting eligibility of the Federal Stafford Loan. Some students, because of other financial aid and other resources, may not qualify for the full amount. The interest is equal to the 91-Day Treasury Bill plus 3%.

HEAL is not subsidized by the federal government. Therefore, the borrower is responsible for interest accrued during enrollment and during any grace or deferment periods. Students may apply for up to $20,000 a year for a four-year total of $80,000.

NATIONAL HEALTH SERVICES CORPS SCHOLARSHIP PROGRAM (NHSC)

NHSC scholarships provide money for tuition, fees, books, supplies, equipment, and a monthly stipend for up to four years of medical school. The following criteria are used to determine eligibility:

1. Be a U.S. citizen attending a U.S. medical school.

2. Preference is given to students interested in primary health care specialties.

3. Preference is given to prior NHSC recipients and disadvantaged backgrounds.

Applicants who are considered will be interviewed and, if they accept, agree to serve one year of full-time clinical primary health care services for each year of support. The minimum obligation is two years. For more information, students can get applications fro their financial aid office or by writing to: NHSC Scholarship Program, 8201 Greensboro Drive, Suite 600, McLean, VA 22102-9975, (800) 221-9393 or (703) 734-6855

PRIMARY CARE LOAN (PCL)

Formerly the HPSL (U.S. Health Professions Student Loan), the PCL is a loan designed to increase the number of doctors in the primary care field. Recipients must enter and complete a residency training program in primary health care (family medicine, general pediatrics, general internal medicine, obstetrics-gynecology, general psychiatry) not later than four years after the date on which the student graduates from medical school. Furthermore, the student must practice in the chosen field through the date on which the loan is repaid. Any borrower who fails to complete a primary care residency and/or practice in a primary health care field will have his or her loan balance recomputed from the date of issuance at an interest rate of 12 percent per year instead of the usual 5 percent, compounded annually.

SCHOLARSHIPS FOR STUDENTS OF EXCEPTIONAL FINANCIAL NEED (EFN)

This federally funded program provides grants to students whose resources do not exceed the lesser of $5,000 or one half the cost of their medical education. Grants cover the cost of tuition and all other expenses except for living expenses. The student's financial resources must not exceed the lesser of $5,000 or one half of the cost of the medical education.

Recipients must enter and complete a residency program in a primary care specialty not later than four years after completion of the M.D. degree (see PCL). Students who fail to maintain academic standards and graduates who fail to comply with the primary care requirements will be liable to the federal government for the amount of the EFN award and for any interest on that amount at the maximum legal prevailing rate.

Other Types of Financial Assistance

Besides grants, merit awards, and federal loans based on financial need and/or minority/disadvantaged status, there are other types of financial aid available for medical students. No candidate will ever be turned away because he or she can't afford medical school. The school's financial aid officer should have a list of everything the school offers as well as information about certain types of financial aid not offered directly through the financial aid office. Some other types of financial aid you may want to get information about are:

Medical Student Research Scholarships: Most medical schools have research programs conducted by faculty and staff. Not only do students get valuable experience and a scholarship for participating in research, they often get credit toward their basic sciences.

Funds For In-State Students: Residents should fill out appropriate forms for "state-sponsored" scholarships immediately after being accepted for admission. Sometimes there is a separate financial aid form other than the one completed for other types of financial aid. And since these are limited and given away quickly, you need to get the forms in well before the deadline.

Funds For Combined Degree Programs: Highly qualified and motivated students wishing to spend 6 to 7 years studying for a combined M.D./Ph.D. degree may qualify for funding available specifically for them. Typically, funding for a combined M.D./Ph.D. candidate will be available for up to six years, though the six years need not be consecutive. Other combined degree programs that qualify are: M.D./J.D. degree, M.D./M.P.H. degree, and M.D./M.B.A. degree.

Private Endowments: Though not common, there are some corporations that make funds available directly to students. The majority, though, distribute funds to medical schools which then award these funds to the medical students. If there are some scholarships or grants available through these channels, the financial aid officer will have either the information or the applications.

12

Alternate Health Careers

As much as some students try, they just can't seem to gain admission to a medical school. If you're one of those students, there are many other careers in the health care field that may interest you enough to look into further. Keep in mind, though, that some professional schools such as physicians assistant or physical therapy may be just as difficult to get into. One advisor, in fact, told me that it's easier nowadays to get into medical school than it is to get into a veterinary school, since there are much fewer of those.

If you're set on making health care your career, other than medicine you may be interested in fields such as physicians assistant, chiropractic, optometry, podiatry, or dentistry. All these fields involve that art of diagnosis, treatment, and healing, but they differ in the methods of treatment they use and in their areas of specialty. Here are descriptions of careers in health diagnosis and treatment. You may learn more by sending for information from the addresses given at the end of each description.

Chiropractic

Chiropractic is a system of treatment based on the principle that a person's health is determined largely by the nervous system, and that interference with this system impairs normal functions and lowers resistance to disease. Chiropractors treat their patients primarily by manual manipulation of body parts, especially the spinal column. Because of the emphasis on the spine and its position, most chiropractors use X-rays to determine the source of a patient's pain or difficulty. In addition to manipulation or spinal adjustments, chiropractors also use water, light, massage, ultrasound, electric, and heat therapy. They also prescribe diet, supports, exercise, and rest, but they do not use prescription drugs or surgery. Most state laws specify the types of supplementary treatment permitted in chiropractic.

Almost all chiropractors work in private offices and are usually self-employed. All 50 states and the District of Columbia regulate the practice of chiropractic, and grant licenses to chiropractors who meet certain educational requirements and pass a State Board Examination. Many states have reciprocity agreements that permit chiropractors already licensed in another state to obtain a license without taking an examination. The type of practice permitted and the educational requirements for licensure vary considerably from state to state. In general, though, state licensing boards require the successful completion of a 4-year chiropractic college accredited by the Council on Chiropractic Education. Most states require a specific number of hours of continuing education in order to maintain licensure.

The National Board of Chiropractic Examiners' test, given to fourth-year chiropractic students, is accepted by most state boards in place of a state examination. All United States accredited chiropractic colleges require applicants to have a minimum of 2 years of undergraduate study including courses in English, social sciences, chemistry, biology, and mathematics. You should examine the school's catalogue for details about specific requirements.

Chiropractic colleges emphasize courses in manipulation and spinal adjustments. Many offer a broader curriculum, including courses in subjects such as physiotherapy and nutrition. In most chiropractic colleges, the emphasis during the first 2 years is on classroom and laboratory work in subjects such as anatomy, physiology, and biochemistry, while the last 2 years stress clinical experiences. Students completing chiropractic training earn the degree of Doctor of Chiropractic (D.C.). For more information about chiropractic and a list of the 15 U.S. chiropractic colleges, write to:

Council on Chiropractic Education
3209 Ingersoll Avenue
Des Moines, IA 50312

Dentistry

Dentists examine teeth and tissues of the mouth to diagnose diseases or abnormalities. They take X-rays, fill cavities, straighten teeth, and treat gum diseases. Laboratory work, such as making dentures and inlays, is done by commercial laboratories specializing in that kind of work. Most dentists are general practitioners who provide many types of dental care. About 10 to 20 percent are specialists, the largest group being orthodontists who straighten teeth. The next largest group, oral surgeons, operate on the mouth and jaws. The remainder specialize in pedodontics (dentistry for children), periodontics (treating the gums), endodontics (root canal therapy), public health dentistry, and oral pathology (diseases of the mouth).

A license to practice dentistry is required in all states and the District of Columbia. To qualify for a license, a candidate must graduate from a dental school approved by the American Dental Association and pass written and practical examinations. Most state licenses permit dentists to engage in both general and specialized practice, although in some states a dentist cannot be licensed as a specialist without having 2 or 3 years of graduate education and, in some cases, passing a state examination. In most states, additional education is also necessary, but a specialist's practice is regulated by the dental profession and not by the state licensing authority. To practice in another state, a licensed dentist usually must pass that state's licensing examination. Some states, however, grant licenses to dentists from other states based solely on their credentials.

Dental school admission requirements vary, but in general require a four-year undergraduate degree from an accredited college or university, though applicants with 90 credit hours will be considered, prerequisite courses similar to that of a premedical curriculum, letters of recommendation, interviews, and the Dental Admissions Test (DAT) similar to the MCAT. Both science and non-science majors are encouraged to apply. There are differences in the two entrance exams, especially the visual and spatial perception part. Prospective applicants need to get a DAT book and study the format used and the kinds of questions that will be asked. Like medical schools, state-supported dental schools give preference to residents of their own states. Applicants should complete the AADSAS (American Association of Dental Schools Application Service) forms, which are similar to AMCAS. Fifty out of fifty-five dental schools nationwide use AADSAS to distribute applications.

Like a medical curriculum, dental school consists of a four-year program in which students begin with classroom instruction and laboratory work in basic sciences such as human anatomy, physiology, microbiology, and biochemistry. Courses in preclinical techniques and beginning courses in clinical sciences are also provided at this time. The last two years are spent chiefly in dental clinics treating patients. The degree of Doctor of Dental Surgery (D.D.S.) is awarded by most dental schools, and an equivalent degree, Doctor of Dental Medicine (D.M.D.) is conferred by some. For additional information about requirements, the DAT, and a list of accredited dental schools write to:

American Association of Dental Schools
1625 Massachusetts Avenue
Washington, DC 20036-2212
(202) 667-9433 or (800) 353-2237

Optometry

Half the people in the United States wear glasses or contact lenses. Optometrists provide much of the vision care these people need. They examine patient's eyes to detect vision problems, diagnose and manage diseases such as glaucoma, cataracts, and retinal disorders, and prescribe eyeglasses and contact lenses, vision aids and eye medications. Typically, when an optometrist detects any sort of disease, he or she would refer the patient to an appropriate health care provider like an ophthalmologist, who is a medical doctor specializing in the eye and eye diseases.

Though most optometrists are in general practice, some specialize in work with children or the elderly, or they concentrate on working with contact lenses or vision therapy. They may work in private practice, multidisciplinary practice, hospitals, research or health centers, public health, or government. Some work for other optometrists or for an ophthalmologist. Once they've finished examining their patients, optometrists will either refer the patient to a physician, prescribe a treatment, or prescribe lenses, which are then made by an optician.

Optometrists are required to complete a four-year degree at one of the 17 accredited U.S. schools of optometry. The prerequisites are basically the same as they are for premed students, except that optometry school applicants take the Optometry Admission Test (OAT) instead of the MCAT. Competition is keen, since there are only a few schools in the nation.

Applicants should also know that there is no clearinghouse service like AMCAS to distribute applications as there is for medical schools and, therefore, each optometry school needs to receive an application separately. The four-year curriculum includes similar courses to medical school but also includes specialized coursework that emphasizes the science of light and vision, lens design and construction, ocular pharmacology, and other vision-related courses.

All states and the District of Columbia require that optometrists be licensed by passing a state board examination. They may also spend a year or more in optometric specialties like family practice optometry, pediatric optometry, low vision rehabilitation, neurooptometry, and low vision rehabilitation. For additional information about optometry and a list of accredited optometry schools, write to:

American Optometric Association
243 North Lindbergh
St. Louis, MO 63141
(314) 991-4100

Osteopathic Medicine

Osteopathic physicians (D.O.s) diagnose and treat diseases or maladies of the human body and place special emphasis on the musculo-skeletal system of the body - i.e. bones, muscles, ligaments, and their associated nerves. About 10 percent of all U.S. physicians are Doctors of Osteopathic Medicine, trained in the same way as M.D.s to do basically everything that M.D.s do. D.O.s also use surgery, drugs, and all other accepted methods of medical care. The majority of osteopathic physicians practice in California, Florida, Illinois, Michigan, Ohio, Kansas, Pennsylvania, New Jersey, Texas, and Missouri.

The major difference between physicians and osteopathic physicians is that the latter are mostly "primary care physicians" who engage in general practice. In recent years, though, more D.O.s have begun to specialize in internal medicine, neurology and psychiatry, ophthalmology, anesthesiology, physical medicine and rehabilitation, dermatology, pathology, radiology, and surgery. Many D.O.s also use osteopathic hospitals exclusively.

Potential osteopathic students need to prepare by taking the same coursework as would be required for premedical students. The osteopathic curriculum is essentially identical to that of medical school, but with more emphasis on primary care and manipulative therapy, which is the main focus of osteopathic medicine. The first half of training involves study in the basic sciences such as anatomy, physiology, and pathology, the remainder devoted largely to experience with patients in hospitals and clinics. Following graduation, nearly all D.O.s serve a 12-month internship (including surgery, pediatrics, internal medicine, and other specialties) at one of the osteo-pathic hospitals approved by the American Osteopathic Association. Those who wish to specialize must have an additional 2 to 5 years of training.

Similar to the AMCAS application that medical school applicants use, applicants to osteopathic schools complete the form used by the American Association of Colleges of Osteopathic Medicine Application Service (AACOMAS). The procedure is identical to AMCAS. Prospective students must also submit letters of recommendation, take the MCAT, and sit for an interview.

All states and the District of Columbia require a license to practice osteopathic medicine. For additional information and a list of the 16 accredited osteopathic schools in the United States, write to:

American Association of Colleges of Osteopathic Medicine
5550 Friendship Blvd.
Suite 310
Chevy Chase, MD 20815-7231
(301) 968-4100

Physician Assistant

With rapid growth in the health care field, more and more hospitals and HMOs are depending on physicians assistants to help provide quality health care. The majority of PAs work in primary care, especially in underserved rural areas and inner cities where traditionally there are few physicians. More recently, however, PAs have become increasingly involved in virtually every medical specialty and subspecialty. And according to the U.S. Department of Labor, there will be nearly a 60 percent increase in the number of PA positions by end of the decade, making this field one of the fastest growing in the health care industry.

Currently there are 60 U.S. programs offering the PA. The majority of applicants accepted hold a four-year college degree, but most schools will consider any applicant who has a minimum of three years at an accredited college or university, so long as they have completed required courses such as biology, chemistry, anatomy & physiology, microbiology, or any other courses a particular school feels are necessary. Other requirements usually include clinical experience. The physician assistant program at Wake Forest University School of Medicine, for example, requires that applicants have six months of full-time employment or 1000 hours of hands-on health care experience. There is no centralized service such as AMCAS for PA school applicants and, therefore, students need to apply to each school individually.

The physician assistant curriculum typically includes both classroom and clinical instruction. The first year is spent studying medical sciences such as anatomy, physiology, pharmacology, laboratory medicine, emergency medical training, and physical assessment. The second year is spent in the clinical setting, where students participate in patient care and serve in clerkships. Students wanting more information on individual programs should write directly to the school. For general information and a list of PA programs throughout the United States, write to:

Association of Physician Assistant Programs
950 N. Washington Street
Alexandria, VA 22314-1552
(703) 548-5538

Podiatry

To get relief from painful feet, a growing number of foot sufferers are paying a visit to the podiatrist. Podiatrists diagnose and treat diseases and deformities of the foot and ankles such as bunions, corns, calluses, ingrown toenails, skin and nail diseases, deformed toes, and arch disabilities. They perform surgery, fit corrective devices, and prescribe drugs, physical therapy, and proper shoes. There is little medical practice in the strict sense of the word. Whenever podiatrists find symptoms of a medical disorder that affects other parts of the body - arthritis, diabetes or heart disease, for example - they refer the patient to a physician while still continuing to treat the foot problem.

Most podiatrists are generalists who provide all types of foot care. Some, however, specialize in foot surgery, orthopedics, podopediatrics (children's foot ailments), or podogeriatrics (foot problems of the elderly). As sports such as jogging, tennis, and racquetball grow in popularity, the specialty of sports medicine is also beginning to show some growth in podiatry.

The D.P.M. degree requires four years of training at one of only 7 accredited schools of podiatric medicine in the United States. Schools use the service provided by the American Association of Colleges of Podiatric Medicine (AACPM) to distribute applications, much like AMCAS does for medical schools. Admission requirements include at least three years or ninety semester hours of college credit, though most accepted students have a bachelor's degree, the same science prerequisites as premed students, the MCAT, extracurricular activities, letters of recommendation, and a personal interview.

The first two years of a podiatric curriculum consists of classroom instruction and laboratory work in anatomy, bacteriology, chemistry, pathology, physiology, pharmacology, and other basic sciences. During the final two years, students gain clinical experience while continuing their academic studies. Additional education and experience are necessary to practice in a specialty.

Following graduation, students must pass a state licensing examination in order to practice. Some states require graduates to serve a one-year residency in a hospital or clinic following graduation. Most states grant licenses without further examination to podiatrists already licensed in another state. For more information and a list of podiatric colleges, write to:

American Association of Colleges of Podiatric Medicine
6110 Executive Blvd.
Suite 204
Rockville, MD 20852
(301) 984-9350 or (800) 922-9266

Veterinary Medicine

The doctor who treats animals rather than people, the government official who inspects meat sold at the supermarket, the scientist who heads a medical research team investigating the mysteries of disease - any one of these could be a veterinarian or Doctor of Veterinary Medicine (D.V.M.). Veterinarians diagnose, treat, and control animal diseases and injuries. They help prevent the outbreak and spread of animal diseases, some of which can easily be transmitted to human beings, perform surgery on sick and injured animals, and prescribe and administer medicines and vaccines. Most veterinarians treat small animals and/or pets exclusively. Some specialize in such fields as the health and breeding of cattle, poultry, sheep, swine, or horses. Others work in laboratories as part of federal and state public health programs.

Students interested in this field should prepare differently than students planning a career in medicine or dentistry. For one thing, competition for vet school is extremely keen, maybe even more so than for medical school. Since there are only 27 veterinary schools in the U.S., it's rare for a student to be accepted at any out-of-state school. Pre-veterinary students need to work extra hard at getting involved with veterinarians as soon as possible; doing volunteer work, spending summers working at vet clinics, doing veterinary research, and working for several different veterinarians during the undergraduate years.

Applicants to vet schools follow the same basic prerequisites as premed students, but they take the Veterinary College Admission Test (VCAT). A few schools will take the Graduate Record Exam Advanced Test in Biology (GRE) or the MCAT. Other requirements include a high GPA, letters of recommendation, and several years of experience with animals and veterinarians. Applicants need to read the prerequisites for the individual school for specific admissions criteria. Recently, more women nationwide have been applying to veterinary schools than men. In the South and West, regional educational plans permit cooperating states without any veterinary colleges to send students to designated regional schools. In other areas, colleges that accept out-of-state students give priority to applicants from nearby states that don't have veterinary schools.

All states require veterinarians to have a license. Graduates take a state board proficiency examination, and some states will issue licenses without further examination to veterinarians already licensed by another state. For research or teaching positions, an additional master's or Ph.D. degree is usually required in a field such as pathology, physiology, toxicology, or laboratory animal medicine. For more information about veterinary medicine, career opportunities, and a list of U.S. veterinary schools write to:

American Veterinary Medicine Association
1931 North Meacham Road
Suite 100
Schaumburg, IL 60173
(847) 925-8070

Other Health-Related Careers

The health careers already discussed are the most popular alternatives for premedical students who decide on another option other than medical school. The following brief descriptions of other health careers are also an alternative, but they don't require the same admission standards and the same extensive professional training as, say, medical or dental school. They do, however, provide a challenging and rewarding lifetime career. Each area is listed in alphabetical order.

Audiologist: Audiologists are specially trained to treat individuals with impaired hearing and vestibular problems (problems of balance and equilibrium). They are responsible for preventing hearing loss and identifying and rehabilitating those who have impaired hearing. By utilizing special instruments, audiologists can identify specific problems and assist in improving whatever hearing remains. Applicants must complete a 4-year college degree, then go on for one of many different advanced degree such as M.S., Ph.D., Ed.D. or Au.D, which is the doctor of audiology. Graduates find employment at hospitals, clinics, colleges and universities, state and federal agencies, industry, rehabilitation centers, and nursing homes. Some go into private practice, others work with physicians. For more information about career opportunities, write to: Audiology Foundation of America, 207 North Street Suite 103, West Lafayette, IN 47906-3083, (765) 743-6283

Dietitian/Nutritionist: Dietitians and nutritionists provide nutritional counseling to individuals and groups, set up and supervise food service systems for institutions such as hospitals, schools, nursing homes, and clinics, and promote sound eating habits through public education and/or research. They often work for federal government, corporations, or city and state agencies. With more people becoming increasingly diet and health conscious, dietitians are even setting up their own consulting firms and starting their own businesses. For more information about a career as a dietitian, write to: American Dietetic Association 216 West Jackson Blvd. Chicago, IL 60606-6995, (312) 899-0040

Health Administrator: Health administrators are more business people than they are scientists. In fact, the Master of Health Administration or Master of Hospital Administration (M.H.A.) is a business degree requiring the applicant to take the Graduate Record Examination (GRE) or the Graduate Management Admission Test (GMAT) for entrance. The undergraduate major may be in any field, but a background in accounting, finance, or business administration is helpful and desirable. Following graduation, health administrators may work for hospitals, clinics, colleges and universities, the school system, or private practice. Programs at 45 U.S. schools typically require two years beyond the bachelor's degree. For more information about Health Administration, write to: Association of University Programs in Health Administration, 1911 N. Fort Meyer Drive, Suite 503, Arlington, VA 22209, (703) 524-5500, ext. 123

Occupational Therapist: Occupational therapists provide services to people who are mentally, physically, or emotionally disabled. They select activities that are designed to develop independence, prepare patients to return to work, develop or restore basic functions, and aid in adjustment to disabilities. They often work in private practice, hospitals and clinics, or federal and state agencies. A bachelor's degree is a prerequisite for occupational therapy programs. Curricula include basic human sciences, behavioral sciences, and sociology as well as occupational therapy theory and practice, which includes at least six months of supervised clinical experience. For more information, write to: American Occupational Therapy Association, 4720 Montogomery Lane, P.O. Box 31220, Bethesda, MD 20824-1220, (301) 962-2682

Nurse: Nurses observe, assess, and record symptoms, reactions, and progress of patients under their care, administer medications, assist in the rehabilitation of patients, instruct patients and family members in proper health maintenance care, and help maintain a proper physical and emotional environment that promotes recovery. Nursing programs include not only basic science courses such as anatomy, physiology, and microbiology, they include clinical experiences with patients and work at hospitals in order to acquaint the student with medical situations.

Following graduation, nurses may enter different fields such as obstetrics/gynecology, oncology, emergency room nursing, or cardiac care. As much in demand as nurses are, they may find employment not only in hospitals, but in private practice, clinics, nursing homes, home care, and schools. For more information about the nursing profession, write to: Academy of Nursing, 600 Maryland Avenue, S.W., Suite 100 West, Washington, D.C. 20024-2571, (202) 651-7238

Pharmacist: Pharmacists dispense drugs and medicines prescribed by doctors and dentists. They also supply and advise people on the use of drugs and on medicines that can be obtained without prescriptions. Students may become pharmacists by earning a second bachelor's degree in pharmacy or a master's degree in pharmacy. Applicants must take the Pharmacy College Admission Test (PAC) and should have a strong science background, especially in chemistry. For more information and a list of the 79 schools and colleges of pharmacy, write to: American Association of Colleges of Pharmacy, 1426 Prince Street, Alexandria, VA 22314-2841, (703) 739-2330

Physical Therapist: Physical therapists plan and administer treatment for patients referred by a physician in order to restore bodily functions, relieve pain, or prevent permanent disability following a disabling injury or disease. Their patients include accident victims, handicapped adults and children, and stroke victims, as well as individuals suffering from nerve injuries, amputations, fractures, and arthritis. All physical therapists have a bachelor's degree, some a master's or doctorate. Most individuals become physical therapists by earning a second bachelor's degree in physical therapy, which requires and additional two years. The best way to prepare for a curriculum in physical therapy is to take a premedical curriculum.

Currently there are 138 accredited physical therapy programs in the United States. Following graduation, students work in hospitals, rehabilitation centers, nursing homes, private practice, or with physicians. Students with a background in athletics may choose to work in sports medicine. Each school has its own admissions criteria, but many are very competitive and may require the Graduate Record Examination (GRE) for entrance. For more information, write to: American Physical Therapy Association, 1111, North Fairfax Street, Alexandria, VA 22314-1488, (703) 684-2782

Public Health Official: Individuals involved in public health deal with the prevention and control of disease, as well as the improvement of health in the community. Students interested in public health may apply to one of 27 accredited schools of public health in the United States. College major is not important, but successful applicants usually have a background in both science and business. Following graduation and awarding of the Master of Public Health (M.P.H.) or Doctor of Public Health (Dr.P.H.), graduates may specialize in one of nine fields: Biostatistics, environmental health, epidemiology, health administration, health education, maternal and child health, parasitology, nutrition, or public health nursing. Employment is mainly in health agencies, government agencies, hospitals, clinics, and research centers. For more information about public health, write to: Association of Schools of Public Health, 1660 L Street, N.W., Suite 204, Washington, DC 20036, (202) 296-1099

Radiology Technologist: Radio technologists or technicians operate radiologic equipment and take X-rays. There are three specialties: X-ray technician, radiation technologist, and nuclear medicine technologist. Students enter a program that includes anatomy, physiology, patient care, physics, radiation protection, imaging, medical terminology, ethics, and pathology. Graduates work mainly in hospitals and clinics, but some are employed by physicians in private practice or federal and state agencies. For additional information about career opportunities in the radiology field, write to: American Society of Radiologic Technologists, 15000 Central Avenue, S.E., Albuquerque, NM 87123-3917, (505) 298-4500

Respiratory Therapist: Respiratory therapists, sometimes called inhalation therapists, treat patients with cardio-pulmonary problems. Responsibilities include treating patients with chronic asthma or emphysema to giving emergency care in cases of heart failure, stroke, drowning, or shock. Typically, respiratory therapists enroll in a program that includes human anatomy and physiology, chemistry, physics, microbiology, and mathematics. Graduates find employment mainly in hospitals and health clinics but more are working for home care services. For more information, write to: American Association for Respiratory Care, 11030 Ables Lane Dallas, TX 75229, (972) 243-2272

Speech Pathologist: Speech pathologists assist people who have communication disorders. They identify, evaluate, and treat individuals with speech problems, as well as prevent those problems through public education and research. Many speech pathologists work for public and private schools, hospitals and clinics, or government agencies. Like audiology applicants, students interested in speech pathology pursue a graduate degree and, in many states, must pass a proficiency test. For more information, write to: American Speech-Language-Hearing Association, 10801 Rockville Pike, Rockville, MD 20852, (301) 897-5700 or (800) 498-2071

Surgical Technician: Surgical technicians, occasionally called surgical technologists or operating room technicians, assist surgeons and anesthesiologists before, during, and after surgery. They always work under the supervision of registered nurses or surgical technologist supervisors. Their main function is to set up operating rooms with the instruments, equipment, sterile linens, and fluids such as glucose that will be needed during an operation. Surgical technicians may also prepare patients for surgery by washing, shaving, and disinfecting body areas where the surgeon will operate. During surgery, they pass instruments and other sterile supplies to the surgeon and the surgeon's assistants.

Professional School Admissions Tests

In order to be accepted as a student in one of the professional schools, you need to take an admissions exam similar to the MCAT. For information about the test, test dates, registration deadlines, etc., write to the following agencies and test services:

DENTAL ADMISSION TESTING PROGRAM (DAT)
> 211 East Chicago Avenue, Suite 1840, Chicago, IL 60611-2678, (800) 621-8099

OPTOMETRY COLLEGE ADMISSION TEST (OAT)
> 211 East Chicago Avenue, Suite 1846, Chicago, IL 60611-2678, (312) 440-2693

PHARMACY COLLEGE ADMISSION TEST (PCAT)
> The Psychological Corporation, 555 Academic Court, San Antonio, TX 78204, (800) 622-3231

VETERINARY COLLEGE ADMISSION TEST (VCAT)
> The Psychological Corporation, 555 Academic Court, San Antonio, TX 78204, (800) 622-3231

MEDICAL COLLEGE ADMISSION TEST (MCAT)
> P.O. Box 4056, Iowa City, IA 52243, (319) 337-1357

Current Health Career Trends

Due to the growth and aging of the U.S. population, overall employment in health care will increase faster than ever. Some fields, however, will experience even faster than average growth because of home and nursing care, and the special services that will be needed specifically by the aging members of the population. The following is a list of the top ten health-related careers that seem to be growing fastest in terms of vacancy rates and employment opportunities. They are listed in the order of greatest opportunities that will be available by the end of the decade and beyond. Students deciding that medicine is not for them may want to consider one of these other options.

1. Occupational Therapy
2. Speech Pathology/Audiology
3. Physical Therapy
4. Physician Assistant
5. Nurse Practitioner
6. Nursing Aide
7. Radiologic Technology
8. Respiratory Therapy
9. Dietitian/Nutritionist
10. Surgical Technician

Appendix A

United States Medical Schools

The following is a complete listing by state and the addresses of all United States medical schools. For detailed information and curriculla information, contact the school directly. Included here are "estimated" annual costs (tuition, books, fees, etc.), the total number of in-state and out-of-state applicants, latest enrollments for both male and female applicants, typical GPAs and MCAT scores of incoming students, and whether the school is public or private. The application deadlines are the latest dates that the school will accept applications. Percent interviewed is the average overall interview rate for both in and out-of-state students.

The actual interview percentage of in-state residents is typically much higher than out-of-state residents. For example, the total percent of applicants interviewed may be 50%, but the percentage of in-state residents interviewed may be 85% versus 15% for out-of-state residents. The chances, therefore, of getting an interview are much greater in your own state of residence. The actual numbers of students interviewed from in and out-of-state may be obtained from the *AAMC Medical School Admissions Requirements.* You should consult the latest school catalogues for any changes in tuition, fees, and other expenses.

ALABAMA

UNIVERSITY OF ALABAMA
School of Medicine
Office of Medical Student Admissions
VH200
Birmingham, AL 35294-0019
In-state applicants: 546; out-of-state applicants: 1,438. Percent interviewed: 55%. First year enrollment: 102 men, women. In-state acceptance rate: 87%. Average GPA: 3.6. Average MCAT score: 9.7. Deadline: Nov 1. Estimated annual cost: residents, $8,500; non-residents, $20,500. Public.

UNIVERSITY OF SOUTH ALABAMA
College of Medicine
Office of Admissions, 2015 MSB
Mobile, AL 36688-0002
In-state applicants: 493; out-of-state applicants: 748. Percent interviewed: 50%. First year enrollment: 39 men, 26 women. In-state acceptance rate: 92%. Average GPA: 3.6. Average MCAT score: 9. Deadline: Nov 15. Estimated annual cost: residents, $9,000; non-residents, $16,000. Public.

ARIZONA

UNIVERSITY OF ARIZONA
College of Medicine
Admissions Office, Room 2209
Tucson, AZ 85724-5075
In-state applicants: 541; out-of-state applicants: 594. Percent interviewed: 50%. First year enrollment: 58 men, 42 women. In-state acceptance rate: 100%. Average GPA: 3.5. Average MCAT score: 9.4. Deadline: Nov 1. Estimated annual cost: residents, $7,500. Public.

ARKANSAS

UNIVERSITY OF ARKANSAS
College of Medicine
Office of Student Admissions, Slot 551
4301 West Markham Street
Little Rock, AR 72205-7199
In-state applicants: 417; out-of-state applicants: 489. Percent interviewed: 70%. First year enrollment: 105 men, 40 women. In-state acceptance rate: 97%. Average GPA: 3.5. Average MCAT score: 7.6. Deadline: Nov 1. Estimated annual cost: residents, $8,000; non-residents, $16,000. Public.

CALIFORNIA

UNIVERSITY OF CALIFORNIA - DAVIS
School of Medicine
Admissions Office
Davis, CA 95616
In-state applicants: 3,819; out-of-state applicants: 788. Percent interviewed: 20%. First year enrollment: 50 men, 43 women. In-state acceptance rate: 99%. Average GPA: 3.5. Average MCAT score: 11. Deadline: Nov 1. Estimated annual cost: residents, $9,000; non-residents, $18,000. Public.

UNIVERSITY OF CALIFORNIA - IRVINE
College of Medicine
P.O. Box 4089
Medical Education Building
Irvine, CA 92717
In-state applicants: 3,839; out-of-state applicants: 427. Percent interviewed: 20%. First year enrollment: 57 men, 35 women. In-state acceptance rate: 99%. Average GPA: 3.5. Average MCAT score: 10.2. Deadline: Nov 1. Estimated annual cost: residents, $9,000; non-residents, $18,000. Public.

UNIVERSITY OF CALIFORNIA - LOS ANGELES
School of Medicine
Division of Admissions
Center for Health Sciences
Los Angeles, CA 90095-1720
In-state applicants: 5,155; out-of-state applicants: 2,146. Percent interviewed: 12%. First year enrollment: 87 men, 72 women. In-state acceptance rate: 89%. Average GPA: 3.6. Average MCAT score: 10.7. Deadline: Nov 1. Estimated annual cost: residents, $9,000; non-residents, $18,000. Public.

DREW/UCLA JOINT MEDICAL PROGRAM
Drew University of Medicine and Science
1621 East 120th Street
Los Angeles, CA 90059

In-state applicants: NA; out-of-state applicants: NA. Percent interviewed: NA. First year enrollment: NA men, NA women. In-state acceptance rate: 90%. Average GPA: NA. Average MCAT score: NA. Deadline: Nov 15. Estimated annual cost: residents, $9,000; non-residents, $18,000. Public.

UNIVERSITY OF CALIFORNIA - SAN DIEGO
School of Medicine
Office of Admissions, 0621
9500 Gilman Drive
La Jolla, CA 92093-0621
In-state applicants: 3,626; out-of-state applicants: 1,241. Percent interviewed: 16%. First year enrollment: 72 men, 50 women. In-state acceptance rate: 98%. Average GPA: 3.6. Average MCAT score: 11. Deadline: Nov 1. Estimated annual cost: residents, $9,000; non-residents, $18,000. Public.

UNIVERSITY OF CALIFORNIA - SAN FRANCISCO
School of Medicine
Admissions, C - 200, Box 0408
San Francisco, CA 94143
In-state applicants: 2,871; out-of-state applicants: 2,660. Percent interviewed: 15%. First year enrollment: 63 men, 90 women. In-state acceptance rate: 77%. Average GPA: 3.7. Average MCAT score: 11. Deadline: Nov 1. Estimated annual cost: residents, $9,000; non-residents, $17,000. Public.

LOMA LINDA UNIVERSITY
School of Medicine
Associate Dean for Admissions
Loma Linda, CA 92350
In-state applicants: 2,129; out-of-state applicants: 2,155. Percent interviewed: 45%. First year enrollment: 95 men, 63 women. In-state acceptance rate: 56%. Average GPA: 3.6. Average MCAT score: 8.9. Deadline: Nov 15. Estimated annual cost: residents, $24,000; non-residents, $24,000. Private.

UNIVERSITY OF SOUTHERN CALIFORNIA
School of Medicine
Office of Admissions
1975 Zonal Avenue
Los Angeles, CA 90033
In-state applicants: 3,686; out-of-state applicants: 2,488. Percent interviewed: 22%. First year enrollment: 89 men, 61 women. In-state acceptance rate: 82%. Average GPA: 3.5. Average MCAT score: 10. Deadline: Nov 1. Estimated annual cost: residents, $29,000; non-residents, $29,000. Private.

STANFORD UNIVERSITY
School of Medicine
Office of Admissions
851 Welch Road, Room 154
Palo Alto, CA 94304-1677

In-state applicants: 2,455; out-of-state applicants: 3,937. Percent interviewed: 10%. First year enrollment: 36 men, 49 women. In-state acceptance rate: 52%. Average GPA: 3.6. Average MCAT score: 11. Deadline: Nov 1. Estimated annual cost: residents, $26,000; non-residents, $26,000. Private.

COLORADO

UNIVERSITY OF COLORADO
School of Medicine
Medical School Admissions
4200 East 9th Avenue, C-297
Denver, CO 80262
In-state applicants: 709; out-of-state applicants: 1,745. Percent interviewed: 55%. First year enrollment: 62 men, 69 women. In-state acceptance rate: 79%. Average GPA: 3.7. Average MCAT score: 9.9. Deadline: Nov 15. Estimated annual cost: residents, $12,500; non-residents, $52,000. Public.

CONNECTICUT

UNIVERSITY OF CONNECTICUT
School of Medicine
Office of Admissions and Student Affairs
263 Farmington Avenue, Room AG-062
Farmington, CT 06030-1950
In-state applicants: 427; out-of-state applicants: 2,311. Percent interviewed: 32%. First year enrollment: 37 men, 46 women. In-state acceptance rate: 90%. Average GPA: 3.5. Average MCAT score: 9.7. Deadline: Dec 15. Estimated annual cost: residents, $12,000; non-residents, $23,000. Public.

YALE UNIVERSITY
School of Medicine
Office of Admissions
367 Cedar Street
New Haven, CT 06510
In-state applicants: 148; out-of-state applicants: 3,368. Percent interviewed: 25%. First year enrollment: 56 men, 45 women. In-state acceptance rate: 10%. Average GPA: 3.6. Average MCAT score: 11.2. Deadline: Oct 15. Estimated annual cost: residents, $25,000; non-residents, $25,000. Private.

DISTRICT OF COLUMBIA

GEORGE WASHINGTON UNIVERSITY
School of Medicine and Health Sciences
Office of Admissions
2300 Eye Street, NW, Room 615
Washington, DC 20037
In-state applicants: 493; out-of-state applicants: 9,360. Percent interviewed: 20%. First year enrollment: 84 men, 69 women. In-state acceptance rate: 6%. Average GPA: 3.5. Average MCAT score: 9.4. Deadline: Dec 1. Estimated annual cost: residents, $31,000; non-residents, $31,000. Private.

GEORGETOWN UNIVERSITY

School of Medicine

Office of Admissions

3900 Reservoir Road, NW

Washington, DC 20007

In-state applicants: 386; out-of-state applicants: 9,254. Percent interviewed: 26%. First year enrollment: 91 men, 70 women. In-state acceptance rate: 3%. Average GPA: 3.5. Average MCAT score: 10.0. Deadline: Nov 1. Estimated annual cost: residents, $25,000; non-residents, $25,000. Private.

HOWARD UNIVERSITY

College of Medicine

Admissions Office

520 W Street, NW

Washington, DC 20059

In-state applicants: 496; out-of-state applicants: 5,017. Percent interviewed: 11%. First year enrollment: 60 men, 59 women. In-state acceptance rate: 6%. Average GPA: 3.0. Average MCAT score: 7.0. Deadline: Dec 15. Estimated annual cost: residents, $17,000; non-residents, $17,000. Private.

FLORIDA

FLORIDA STATE UNIVERSITY

Program in Medical Sciences

Tallahassee, FL 32306-4051

In-state applicants: NA; out-of-state applicants: NA. Percent interviewed: NA. First year enrollment: men, NA women, NA. In-state acceptance rate: 99%. Average GPA: NA. Average MCAT score: NA. Deadline: Dec 1. Estimated annual cost: residents, $9,000; non-residents, $23,000. Public.

UNIVERSITY OF FLORIDA

College of Medicine

J. Hillis Miller Health Center

Gainesville, FL 32610

In-state applicants: 1,860; out-of-state applicants: 1,571. Percent interviewed: 20%. First year enrollment: 57 men, 57 women. In-state acceptance rate: 99%. Average GPA: 3.7. Average MCAT score: 9.3. Deadline: Dec 1. Estimated annual cost: residents, $9,000; non-residents, $23,000. Public.

UNIVERSITY OF MIAMI

School of Medicine

Office of Admissions

P.O. Box 016159

Miami, FL 33101

In-state applicants: 1,292; out-of-state applicants: 1,211. Percent interviewed: 70%. First year enrollment: 70 men, 71 women. In-state acceptance rate: 99%. Average GPA: 3.6. Average MCAT score: 9.4. Deadline: Dec 1. Estimated annual cost: residents, $24,000; non-residents, $29,000. Private.

UNIVERSITY OF SOUTH FLORIDA

College of Medicine

Office of Admissions, Box 3

12901 Bruce B. Downs Blvd.

Tampa, FL 33612-4799

In-state applicants: 1,026; out-of-state applicants: 313. Percent interviewed: 45%. First year enrollment: 61 men, 35 women. In-state acceptance rate: 99%. Average GPA: 3.7. Average MCAT score: 9.7. Deadline: Dec 1. Estimated annual cost: residents, $9,000; non-residents, $23,000. Public.

GEORGIA

EMORY UNIVERSITY

School of Medicine

Administration Building, Admissions, Room 303

Atlanta, GA 30322-4510

In-state applicants: 660; out-of-state applicants: 7,105. Percent interviewed: 20%. First year enrollment: 66 men, 46 women. In-state acceptance rate: 55%. Average GPA: 3.6. Average MCAT score: 9.8. Deadline: Oct 15. Estimated annual cost: residents, $23,000; non-residents, $23,000. Private.

MEDICAL COLLEGE OF GEORGIA

School of Medicine

Associate Dean for Admissions

Augusta, GA 30912-4760

In-state applicants: 917; out-of-state applicants: 747. Percent interviewed: 27%. First year enrollment: 129 men, 51 women. In-state acceptance rate: 99%. Average GPA: 3.5. Average MCAT score: 9.5. Deadline: Nov 1. Estimated annual cost: residents, $6,000; non-residents, $19,000. Public.

MERCER UNIVERSITY

School of Medicine

Office of Admissions and Student Affairs

Macon, GA 31207

In-state applicants: 690; out-of-state applicants: 525. Percent interviewed: 22%. First year enrollment: 37 men, 18 women. In-state acceptance rate: 100%. Average GPA: 3.5. Average MCAT score: 9.4. Deadline: Dec 1. Estimated annual cost: residents, $19,000. Private.

MOREHOUSE SCHOOL OF MEDICINE

Admissions and Student Affairs

720 Westview Drive, SW

Atlanta, GA 30310-1495

In-state applicants: 367; out-of-state applicants: 2,456. Percent interviewed: 10%. First year enrollment: 13 men, 22 women. In-state acceptance rate: 53%. Average GPA: 3.0. Average MCAT score: 7.0. Deadline: Dec 1. Estimated annual cost: residents, $18,500; non-residents, $18,500. Private.

HAWAII

UNIVERSITY OF HAWAII
John A. Burns School of Medicine
Office of Admissions
1960 East - West Road
Honolulu, HI 96822
In-state applicants: 227; out-of-state applicants: 1,001. Percent interviewed: 27%. First year enrollment: 34 men, 31 women. In-state acceptance rate: 80%. Average GPA: 3.4. Average MCAT score: 9.5. Deadline: Dec 1. Estimated annual cost: residents, $9,500; non-residents, $23,000. Public.

ILLINOIS

UNIVERSITY OF CHICAGO
Pritzker School of Medicine
Office of the Dean of Students
924 East 57th Street, BLSC 104
Chicago, IL 60637
In-state applicants: 1,177; out-of-state applicants: 7,055. Percent interviewed: 22%. First year enrollment: 60 men, 44 women. In-state acceptance rate: 49%. Average GPA: 3.5. Average MCAT score: 10.2. Deadline: Nov 15. Estimated annual cost: residents, $23,000; non-residents, $23,000. Private.

FINCH UNIVERSITY OF HEALTH SCIENCES / CHICAGO MEDICAL SCHOOL
Office of Admissions
3333 Green Bay Road
North Chicago, IL 60064
In-state applicants: 1,345; out-of-state applicants: 9,866. Percent interviewed: 15%. First year enrollment: 107 men, 73 women. In-state acceptance rate: 42%. Average GPA: 3.2. Average MCAT score: 9.0. Deadline: Dec 15. Estimated annual cost: residents, $30,000; non-residents, $30,000. Private.

UNIVERSITY OF ILLINOIS
College of Medicine
Office of Medical College Admissions
808 South Wood Street
Chicago, IL 60612-7302
In-state applicants: 1,926; out-of-state applicants: 2,639. Percent interviewed: 30%. First year enrollment: 166 men, 106 women. In-state acceptance rate: 92%. Average GPA: 3.4. Average MCAT score: 9.3. Deadline: Dec 15. Estimated annual cost: residents, $12,000; non-residents, $34,000. Public.

LOYOLA UNIVERSITY
Stritch School of Medicine
Office of Admissions, Room 1752
2160 South First Avenue
Maywood, IL 60153

In-state applicants: 1,622; out-of-state applicants: 7,492. Percent interviewed: 12%. First year enrollment: 68 men, 62 women. In-state acceptance rate: 50%. Average GPA: 3.5. Average MCAT score: 9.5. Deadline: Nov 15. Estimated annual cost: residents, $28,000; non-residents, $28,000. Private.

NORTHWESTERN UNIVERSITY

Medical School

Associate Dean for Admissions

303 East Chicago Avenue

Chicago, IL 60611

In-state applicants: 1,290; out-of-state applicants: 7,425. Percent interviewed: 10%. First year enrollment: 94 men, 80 women. In-state acceptance rate: 35%. Average GPA: 3.5. Average MCAT score: 9.7. Deadline: Oct 15. Estimated annual cost: residents, $28,000; non-residents, $28,000. Private.

RUSH MEDICAL COLLEGE

Office of Admissions

524 Academic Facility

600 South Paulina Street

Chicago, IL 60612

In-state applicants: 1,685; out-of-state applicants: 3,531. Percent interviewed: 20%. First year enrollment: 70 men, 50 women. In-state acceptance rate: 83%. Average GPA: 3.4. Average MCAT score: 9.1. Deadline: Nov 15. Estimated annual cost: residents, $25,000; non-residents, $25,000. Private.

SOUTHERN ILLINOIS UNIVERSITY

School of Medicine

Office of Student and Alumni Affairs

P.O. Box 19230

Springfield, IL 62794-9230

In-state applicants: 1,285; out-of-state applicants: 532. Percent interviewed: 25%. First year enrollment: 46 men, 26 women. In-state acceptance rate: 99%. Average GPA: 3.5. Average MCAT score: 8.8. Deadline: Nov 15. Estimated annual cost: residents, $8,500; non-residents, $23,000. Public.

INDIANA

INDIANA UNIVERSITY

School of Medicine

Medical School Admissions Office

Fesler Hall 213

1120 South Drive

Indianapolis, IN 46202-5113

In-state applicants: 681; out-of-state applicants: 1,629. Percent interviewed: 55%. First year enrollment: 172 men, 108 women. In-state acceptance rate: 91%. Average GPA: 3.6. Average MCAT score: 9.4. Deadline: Dec 15. Estimated annual cost: residents, $12,000; non-residents, $26,500. Public.

IOWA

UNIVERSITY OF IOWA
College of Medicine
Director of Admissions
100 Medicine Administration Building
Iowa City, IA 52242-1101
In-state applicants: 399; out-of-state applicants: 2,007. Percent interviewed: 13%. First year enrollment: 106 men, 69 women. In-state acceptance rate: 78%. Average GPA: 3.6. Average MCAT score: 9.4. Deadline: Nov 1. Estimated annual cost: residents, $10,000; non-residents, $24,000. Public.

KANSAS

UNIVERSITY OF KANSAS
School of Medicine
Associate Dean for Admissions
3901 Rainbow Blvd.
Kansas City, KS 66160-7301
In-state applicants: 420; out-of-state applicants: 1,150. Percent interviewed: 34%. First year enrollment: 103 men, 73 women. In-state acceptance rate: 91%. Average GPA: 3.5. Average MCAT score: 9.1. Deadline: Oct 15. Estimated annual cost: residents, $9,000; non-residents, $22,000. Public.

KENTUCKY

UNIVERSITY OF KENTUCKY
College of Medicine
Chandler Medical Center
800 Rose Street
Lexington, KY 40536-0084
In-state applicants: 508; out-of-state applicants: 1,032. Percent interviewed: 20%. First year enrollment: 60 men, 38 women. In-state acceptance rate: 93%. Average GPA: 3.4. Average MCAT score: 9.0. Deadline: Nov 1. Estimated annual cost: residents, $9,000; non-residents, $20,000. Public.

UNIVERSITY OF LOUISVILLE
School of Medicine
Office of Admissions
Health Sciences Center
Louisville, KY 40292
In-state applicants: 509; out-of-state applicants: 1,227. Percent interviewed: 32%. First year enrollment: 71 men, 66 women. In-state acceptance rate: 91%. Average GPA: 3.4. Average MCAT score: 8.9. Deadline: Nov 1. Estimated annual cost: residents, $8,500; non-residents, $20,000. Public.

LOUISIANA

LOUISIANA STATE UNIVERSITY - NEW ORLEANS
School of Medicine Admissions Office
1901 Perdido Street, Box P3-4
New Orleans, LA 70112-1393
In-state applicants: 705; out-of-state applicants: 521. Percent interviewed: 42%. First year enrollment: 125 men, 64 women. In-state acceptance rate: 99%. Average GPA: 3.4. Average MCAT score: 8.6. Deadline: Nov 15. Estimated annual cost: residents, $7,000; non-residents, $15,000. Public.

LOUISIANA STATE UNIVERSITY - SHREVEPORT
School of Medicine
Office of Admissions
P.O. Box 33932
Shreveport, LA 71130-3932
In-state applicants: 727; out-of-state applicants: 246. Percent interviewed: 25%. First year enrollment: 69 men, 31 women. In-state acceptance rate: 98%. Average GPA: 3.4. Average MCAT score: 8.8. Deadline: Nov 15. Estimated annual cost: residents, $7,000; non-residents, $15,000. Public.

TULANE UNIVERSITY
School of Medicine
Office of Admissions
1430 Tulane Avenue, SL67
New Orleans, LA 70112-2699
In-state applicants: 589; out-of-state applicants: 8,906. Percent interviewed: 13%. First year enrollment: 78 men, 72 women. In-state acceptance rate: 21%. Average GPA: 3.5. Average MCAT score: 9.5. Deadline: Dec 15. Estimated annual cost: residents, $28,000; non-residents, $28,000. Private.

MARYLAND

JOHNS HOPKINS UNIVERSITY
School of Medicine
Committee on Admissions
720 Rutland Avenue
Baltimore, MD 21205-2196
In-state applicants: 335; out-of-state applicants: 3,389. Percent interviewed: 20%. First year enrollment: 62 men, 57 women. In-state acceptance rate: 15%. Average GPA: 3.7. Average MCAT score: 11.3. Deadline: Nov 1. Estimated annual cost: residents, $25,000; non-residents, $25,000. Private.

UNIVERSITY OF MARYLAND
School of Medicine
Committee on Admissions, Room 1-005
655 West Baltimore Street
Baltimore, MD 21201

In-state applicants: 1,030; out-of-state applicants: 3,091. Percent interviewed: 30%. First year enrollment: 77 men, 67 women. In-state acceptance rate: 88%. Average GPA: 3.6. Average MCAT score: 9.8. Deadline: Nov 1. Estimated annual cost: residents, $13,000; non-residents, $23,500. Public.

UNIFORMED SERVICES UNIVERSITY OF THE HEALTH SCIENCES

F. Edward Hebert School of Medicine

Admissions Office, Room A-1041

4301 Jones Bridge Road

Bethesda, MD 20814-4799

In-state applicants: NA; out-of-state applicants: NA. Percent interviewed: NA%. First year enrollment: 127 men, 38 women. In-state acceptance rate: NA%. Average GPA: 3.4. Average MCAT score: 9.8. Deadline: Nov 1. Estimated annual cost: residents, $0; non-residents, $0. Federal.

MASSACHUSETTS

BOSTON UNIVERSITY

School of Medicine Admissions Office

80 East Concord Street

Boston, MA 02118

In-state applicants: 776; out-of-state applicants: 9,856. Percent interviewed: 14%. First year enrollment: 93 men, 58 women. In-state acceptance rate: 25%. Average GPA: 3.3. Average MCAT score: 9.1. Deadline: Nov 15. Estimated annual cost: residents, $32,000; non-residents, $32,000. Private.

HARVARD MEDICAL SCHOOL

Office of Admissions

25 Shattuck Street

Boston, MA 02115-6092

In-state applicants: 311; out-of-state applicants: 3,397. Percent interviewed: 32%. First year enrollment: 92 men, 73 women. In-state acceptance rate: 11%. Average GPA: 3.7. Average MCAT score: 11.5. Deadline: Oct 15. Estimated annual cost: residents, $26,000; non-residents, $26,000. Private.

UNIVERSITY OF MASSACHUSETTS MEDICAL SCHOOL

Associate Dean for Admissions

55 Lake Avenue, North

Worcester, MA 01655

In-state applicants: 778; out-of-state applicants: 587. Percent interviewed: 60%. First year enrollment: 52 men, 48 women. In-state acceptance rate: 100%. Average GPA: 3.5. Average MCAT score: 10.0. Deadline: Nov 1. Estimated annual cost: residents, $10,000. Public.

TUFTS UNIVERSITY

School of Medicine

Office of Admissions

136 Harrison Avenue

Boston, MA 02111

In-state applicants: 760; out-of-state applicants: 9,646. Percent interviewed: 11%. First year enrollment: 108 men, 60 women. In-state acceptance rate: 30%. Average GPA: 3.5. Average MCAT score: 9.2. Deadline: Nov 1. Estimated annual cost: residents, $31,000; non-residents, $31,000. Private.

MICHIGAN

MICHIGAN STATE UNIVERSITY
College of Human Medicine
Office of Admissions
A-239 Life Sciences
East Lansing, MI 48824-1317
(517) 353-9620

In-state applicants: 1,304; out-of-state applicants: 2,271. Percent interviewed: 20%. First year enrollment: 50 men, 56 women. In-state acceptance rate: 86%. Average GPA: 3.4. Average MCAT score: 9.3. Deadline: Nov 15. Estimated annual cost: residents, $15,000; non-residents, $32,000. Public.

UNIVERSITY OF MICHIGAN MEDICAL SCHOOL
Admissions Office
M4130 Medical Sciences Building
Ann Arbor, MI 48109-0611
(734) 764-6317

In-state applicants: 1,113; out-of-state applicants: 4,187. Percent interviewed: 22%. First year enrollment: 100 men, 63 women. In-state acceptance rate: 56%. Average GPA: 3.6. Average MCAT score: 11.1. Deadline: Nov 15. Estimated annual cost: residents, $17,000; non-residents, $26,000. Public.

WAYNE STATE UNIVERSITY
School of Medicine
Director of Admissions
540 East Canfield
Detroit, MI 48201
(313) 577-1466

In-state applicants: 1,495; out-of-state applicants: 2,160. Percent interviewed: 32%. First year enrollment: 145 men, 109 women. In-state acceptance rate: 89%. Average GPA: 3.4. Average MCAT score: 8.9. Deadline: Dec 15. Estimated annual cost: residents, $10,000; non-residents, $20,000. Public.

MINNESOTA

MAYO MEDICAL SCHOOLS
Admissions Committee
200 First Street, SW
Rochester, MN 55905
(507) 284-3671

In-state applicants: 380; out-of-state applicants: 3,241. Percent interviewed: 30%. First year enrollment: 20 men, 22 women. In-state acceptance rate: 21%. Average GPA: 3.6. Average MCAT score: 10.7. Deadline: Nov 1. Estimated annual cost: residents, $20,000; non-residents, $20,000. Private.

UNIVERSITY OF MINNESOTA - DULUTH
School of Medicine
Office of Admissions, Room 107
10 University Drive
Duluth, MN 55812
In-state applicants: 560; out-of-state applicants: 582. Percent interviewed: 42%. First year enrollment: 25 men, 23 women. In-state acceptance rate: 94%. Average GPA: 3.5. Average MCAT score: 9.0. Deadline: Nov 15. Estimated annual cost: residents, $16,000; non-residents, $30,000. Public.

UNIVERSITY OF MINNESOTA
Medical School
Office of Admissions and Student Affairs
420 Delaware Street, SE
Minneapolis, MN 55455-0310
In-state applicants: 829; out-of-state applicants: 1,249. Percent interviewed: 40%. First year enrollment: 91 men, 74 women. In-state acceptance rate: 89%. Average GPA: 3.6. Average MCAT score: 9.7. Deadline: Nov 15. Estimated annual cost: residents, $16,000; non-residents, $30,000. Public.

MISSISSIPPI

UNIVERSITY OF MISSISSIPPI
School of Medicine
Chair, Admissions Committee
2500 North State Street
Jackson, MS 39216-4505
In-state applicants: 309; out-of-state applicants: 296. Percent interviewed: 46%. First year enrollment: 65 men, 35 women. In-state acceptance rate: 99%. Average GPA: 3.6. Average MCAT score: 9.0. Deadline: Nov 1. Estimated annual cost: residents, $7,000; non-residents, $13,000. Public.

MISSOURI

UNIVERSITY OF MISSOURI - COLUMBIA
School of Medicine
Office of Admissions
MA202 Medical Sciences Bldg.
One Hospital Drive
Columbia, MO 65212
In-state applicants: 452; out-of-state applicants: 536. Percent interviewed: 35%. First year enrollment: 54 men, 41 women. In-state acceptance rate: 99%. Average GPA: 3.6. Average MCAT score: 9.3. Deadline: Nov 1. Estimated annual cost: residents, $14,000; non-residents, $27,000. Public.

UNIVERSITY OF MISSOURI - KANSAS CITY
School of Medicine
Admissions Office
2411 Holmes
Kansas City, MO 64108
In-state applicants: 557; out-of-state applicants: 373. Percent interviewed: 60%. First year enrollment: 53 men, 40 women. In-state acceptance rate: 60%. Average GPA: 3.0. Average MCAT score: 8.0. Deadline: Nov 15. Estimated annual cost: residents, $20,000; non-residents, $40,000. Public.

ST. LOUIS UNIVERSITY
School of Medicine
Admissions Committee
1402 South Grand Blvd.
St. Louis, MO 63104
In-state applicants: 382; out-of-state applicants: 6,833. Percent interviewed: 25%. First year enrollment: 81 men, 70 women. In-state acceptance rate: 32%. Average GPA: 3.6. Average MCAT score: 9.9. Deadline: Dec 15. Estimated annual cost: residents, $27,000; non-residents, $27,000. Private.

WASHINGTON UNIVERSITY
School of Medicine
Office of Admissions
660 South Euclid Avenue, #8107
St. Louis, MO 63110
In-state applicants: 215; out-of-state applicants: 5,606. Percent interviewed: 25%. First year enrollment: 60 men, 61 women. In-state acceptance rate: 7%. Average GPA: 3.8. Average MCAT score: 12.0. Deadline: Nov 15. Estimated annual cost: residents, $27,000; non-residents, $27,000. Private.

NEBRASKA

CREIGHTON UNIVERSITY
School of Medicine
Office of Admissions
2500 California Plaza
Omaha, NE 68178
In-state applicants: 280; out-of-state applicants: 5,952. Percent interviewed: 15%. First year enrollment: 58 men, 52 women. In-state acceptance rate: 24%. Average GPA: 3.6. Average MCAT score: 8.8. Deadline: Nov 1. Estimated annual cost: residents, $25,000; non-residents, $25,000. Private.

UNIVERSITY OF NEBRASKA
College of Medicine
Office of Admissions
Wittson Hall, Room 5017A
600 South 42nd Street
Omaha, NE 68198-6585

In-state applicants: 378; out-of-state applicants: 658. Percent interviewed: 40%. First year enrollment: 65 men, 53 women. In-state acceptance rate: 94%. Average GPA: 3.6. Average MCAT score: 9.2. Deadline: Nov 1. Estimated annual cost: residents, $12,000; non-residents, $22,000. Public.

NEVADA

UNIVERSITY OF NEVADA
School of Medicine
Office of Admissions and Student Affairs, Mail Stop 357
Reno, NV 89557
In-state applicants: 162; out-of-state applicants: 956. Percent interviewed: 45%. First year enrollment: 33 men, 19 women. In-state acceptance rate: 90%. Average GPA: 3.4. Average MCAT score: 9.2. Deadline: Nov 1. Estimated annual cost: residents, $9,000; non-residents, $23,000. Public.

NEW HAMPSHIRE

DARTMOUTH MEDICAL SCHOOL
Admissions Office
7020 Remsen, Room 306
Hanover, NH 03755-3833
In-state applicants: 642; out-of-state applicants: 6,494. Percent interviewed: 15%. First year enrollment: men, women. In-state acceptance rate: 12%. Average GPA: 3.5. Average MCAT score: 9.6. Deadline: Nov 1. Estimated annual cost: residents, $25,000; non-residents, $25,000. Private.

NEW JERSEY

UMDNJ - NEW JERSEY MEDICAL SCHOOL
Director of Admissions
185 South Orange Avenue
Newark, NJ 07103
In-state applicants: 1,299; out-of-state applicants: 2,271. Percent interviewed: 34%. First year enrollment: 108 men, 63 women. In-state acceptance rate: 95%. Average GPA: 3.3. Average MCAT score: 9.6. Deadline: Dec 15. Estimated annual cost: residents, $15,000; non-residents, $24,000. Public.

UMDNJ - R.W. JOHNSON MEDICAL SCHOOL
Office of Admissions
675 Hoes Lane
Piscataway, NJ 08854-5635
In-state applicants: 1,316; out-of-state applicants: 2,006. Percent interviewed: 27%. First year enrollment: 74 men, 64 women. In-state acceptance rate: 91%. Average GPA: 3.5. Average MCAT score: 9.4. Deadline: Dec 1. Estimated annual cost: residents, $15,000; non-residents, $24,000. Public.

NEW MEXICO

UNIVERSITY OF NEW MEXICO
School of Medicine
Office of Admissions and Student Affairs
Basic Medical Sciences Bldg., Room 107
Albuquerque, NM 87131-5166
In-state applicants: 322; out-of-state applicants: 857. Percent interviewed: 34%. First year enrollment: 42 men, 31 women. In-state acceptance rate: 96%. Average GPA: 3.5. Average MCAT score: 8.9. Deadline: Nov 15. Estimated annual cost: residents, $5,500; non-residents, $15,500. Public.

NEW YORK

ALBANY MEDICAL COLLEGE
Office of Admissions, A-3
47 New Scotland Avenue
Albany, NY 12208
In-state applicants: 2,056; out-of-state applicants: 6,477. Percent interviewed: 27%. First year enrollment: 69 men, 58 women. In-state acceptance rate: 30%. Average GPA: 3.4. Average MCAT score: 9.9. Deadline: Nov 15. Estimated annual cost: residents, $26,000; non-residents, $28,000. Private.

ALBERT EINSTEIN COLLEGE OF MEDICINE
Office of Admissions
Jack and Pearl Resnick Campus
1300 Morris Park Avenue
Bronx, NY 10461
In-state applicants: 2,049; out-of-state applicants: 6,708. Percent interviewed: 27%. First year enrollment: 91 men, 85 women. In-state acceptance rate: 44%. Average GPA: 3.5. Average MCAT score: 10.0. Deadline: Nov 1. Estimated annual cost: residents, $27,000; non-residents, $27,000. Private.

COLUMBIA UNIVERSITY
College of Physicians and Surgeons
Admissions Office, Room 1-416
630 West 168th Street
New York, NY 10032
In-state applicants: 949; out-of-state applicants: 3,088. Percent interviewed: 40%. First year enrollment: 84 men, 66 women. In-state acceptance rate: 28%. Average GPA: 3.5. Average MCAT score: 11.4. Deadline: Oct 15. Estimated annual cost: residents, $27,000; non-residents, $27,000. Private.

CORNELL UNIVERSITY MEDICAL COLLEGE
Office of Admissions
445 East 69th Street
New York, NY 10021

In-state applicants: 1,498; out-of-state applicants: 5,635. Percent interviewed: 20%. First year enrollment: 47 men, 54 women. In-state acceptance rate: 46%. Average GPA: 3.5. Average MCAT score: 10.8. Deadline: Oct 15. Estimated annual cost: residents, $25,000; non-residents, $25,000. Private.

MOUNT SINAI SCHOOL OF MEDICINE
Director of Admissions Annenberg Bldg., Room 5-04
One Gustave L. Levy Place, Box 1002
New York, NY 10029-6574
In-state applicants: 2,150; out-of-state applicants: 6,122. Percent interviewed: 35%. First year enrollment: 54 men, 51 women. In-state acceptance rate: 48%. Average GPA: 3.4. Average MCAT score: 9.1. Deadline: Nov 1. Estimated annual cost: residents, $22,000; non-residents, $22,000. Private.

NEW YORK MEDICAL COLLEGE
Office of Admissions
Room 127, Sunshine Cottage
Valhalla, NY 10595
In-state applicants: 2,152; out-of-state applicants: 8,826. Percent interviewed: 40%. First year enrollment: 92 men, 92 women. In-state acceptance rate: 27%. Average GPA: 3.3. Average MCAT score: 10.0. Deadline: Dec 1. Estimated annual cost: residents, $27,000; non-residents, $27,000. Private.

NEW YORK UNIVERSITY
School of Medicine Office of Admissions
P.O. Box 1924
New York, NY 10016
In-state applicants: 1,294; out-of-state applicants: 3,213. Percent interviewed: 30%. First year enrollment: 86 men, 73 women. In-state acceptance rate: 48%. Average GPA: 3.6. Average MCAT score: 10.7. Deadline: Dec 1. Estimated annual cost: residents, $25,000; non-residents, $25,000. Private.

UNIVERSITY OF ROCHESTER
School of Medicine and Dentistry
Director of Admissions
Medical Center Box 601
Rochester, NY 14642
In-state applicants: 977; out-of-state applicants: 2,931. Percent interviewed: 23%. First year enrollment: 56 men, 43 women. In-state acceptance rate: 48%. Average GPA: 3.5. Average MCAT score: 8.8. Deadline: Oct 15. Estimated annual cost: residents, $25,000; non-residents, $25,000. Private.

SUNY - BROOKLYN
College of Medicine
Director of Admissions
450 Clarkson Avenue, Box 60M
Brooklyn, NY 11203

In-state applicants: 2,461; out-of-state applicants: 1,607. Percent interviewed: 32%. First year enrollment: 101 men, 79 women. In-state acceptance rate: 99%. Average GPA: 3.5. Average MCAT score: 9.3. Deadline: Dec 15. Estimated annual cost: residents, $11,000; non-residents, $22,000. Public.

UNIVERSITY AT BUFFALO
School of Medicine and Biomedical Sciences
Office of Medical Admissions
40 Biomedical Education Building
Buffalo, NY 14214-3013
In-state applicants: 2,214; out-of-state applicants: 582. Percent interviewed: 22%. First year enrollment: 68 men, 70 women. In-state acceptance rate: 99%. Average GPA: 3.6. Average MCAT score: 9.6. Deadline: Oct 15. Estimated annual cost: residents, $12,000; non-residents, $23,000. Public.

SUNY - STONY BROOK
School of Medicine
Health Sciences Center
Committee on Admissions
Level 4, Room 147
Stony Brook, NY 11794-8434
In-state applicants: 2,507; out-of-state applicants: 831. Percent interviewed: 45%. First year enrollment: 51 men, 49 women. In-state acceptance rate: 99%. Average GPA: 3.5. Average MCAT score: 10.5. Deadline: Nov 15. Estimated annual cost: residents, $11,000; non-residents, $22,000. Public.

SUNY - SYRACUSE
College of Medicine
Admissions Committee
155 Elizabeth Blackwell Street
Syracuse, NY 13210
In-state applicants: 2,319; out-of-state applicants: 752. Percent interviewed: 25%. First year enrollment: 77 men, 70 women. In-state acceptance rate: 99%. Average GPA: 3.5. Average MCAT score: 9.1. Deadline: Nov 1. Estimated annual cost: residents, $11,000; non-residents, $22,000. Public.

NORTH CAROLINA

DUKE UNIVERSITY
School of Medicine
Committee on Admissions
P.O. Box 3710
Durham, NY 27710
In-state applicants: 393; out-of-state applicants: 6,156. Percent interviewed: 35%. First year enrollment: 55 men, 46 women. In-state acceptance rate: 29%. Average GPA: 3.6. Average MCAT score: 11.0. Deadline: Oct 15. Estimated annual cost: residents, $25,000; non-residents, $25,000. Private.

EAST CAROLINA UNIVERSITY

School of Medicine

Office of Admissions

Greenville, NC 27858-4354

In-state applicants: 911; out-of-state applicants: 842. Percent interviewed: 36%. First year enrollment: 38 men, 34 women. In-state acceptance rate: 99%. Average GPA: 3.4. Average MCAT score: 8.0. Deadline: Nov 15. Estimated annual cost: residents, $3,000; non-residents, $22,000. Public.

UNIVERSITY OF NORTH CAROLINA at CHAPEL HILL

School of Medicine

Admissions Office

CB# 7000 MacNider Hall

Chapel Hill, NC 27599-7000

In-state applicants: 956; out-of-state applicants: 1,881. Percent interviewed: 33%. First year enrollment: 75 men, 85 women. In-state acceptance rate: 91%. Average GPA: 3.4. Average MCAT score: 9.0. Deadline: Nov 15. Estimated annual cost: residents, $3,000; non-residents, $23,000. Public.

WAKE FOREST UNIVERSITY SCHOOL OF MEDICINE

(Formerly Bowman Gray School of Medicine)

Office of Medical School Admissions

Medical Center Blvd.

Winston-Salem, NC 27157-1090

In-state applicants: 786; out-of-state applicants: 5,778. Percent interviewed: 15%. First year enrollment: 55 men, 54 women. In-state acceptance rate: 51%. Average GPA: 3.4. Average MCAT score: 9.7. Deadline: Nov 1. Estimated annual cost: residents, $23,000; non-residents, $23,000. Private.

NORTH DAKOTA

UNIVERSITY OF NORTH DAKOTA

School of Medicine

Committee on Admissions

501 North Columbia Road, Box 9037

Grand Forks, ND 58202-9037

In-state applicants: 130; out-of-state applicants: 214. Percent interviewed: 82%. First year enrollment: 28 men, 30 women. In-state acceptance rate: 70%. Average GPA: 3.6. Average MCAT score: 8.7. Deadline: Nov 1. Estimated annual cost: residents, $9,000; non-residents, $23,000. Public.

OHIO

CASE WESTERN RESERVE UNIVERSITY

School of Medicine

Office of Admissions and Student Affairs

10900 Euclid Avenue

Cleveland, OH 44106-4920

In-state applicants: 1,090; out-of-state applicants: 6,228. Percent interviewed: 18%. First year enrollment: 86 men, 58 women. In-state acceptance rate: 62%. Average GPA: 3.5. Average MCAT score: 9.5. Deadline: Oct 15. Estimated annual cost: residents, $25,000; non-residents, $25,000. Private.

UNIVERSITY OF CINCINNATI

School of Medicine Office of Admissions

P.O. Box 670552

Cincinnati, OH 45267-0552

In-state applicants: 1,352; out-of-state applicants: 2,927. Percent interviewed: 18%. First year enrollment: 90 men, 66 women. In-state acceptance rate: 83%. Average GPA: 3.5. Average MCAT score: 9.5. Deadline: Nov 15. Estimated annual cost: residents, $11,500; non-residents, $20,000. Public.

MEDICAL COLLEGE OF OHIO

Admissions Office

P.O. Box 10008

Toledo, OH 43699

In-state applicants: 1,271; out-of-state applicants: 2,912. Percent interviewed: 40%. First year enrollment: 89 men, 51 women. In-state acceptance rate: 81%. Average GPA: 3.4. Average MCAT score: 8.8. Deadline: Nov 1. Estimated annual cost: residents, $11,000; non-residents, $19,000. Public.

NORTHEASTERN OHIO UNIVERSITY

College of Medicine Office of Admissions

P.O. Box 95

Rootstown, OH 44272-0095

In-state applicants: 895; out-of-state applicants: 399. Percent interviewed: 15%. First year enrollment: 56 men, 49 women. In-state acceptance rate: 94%. Average GPA: 3.6. Average MCAT score: 9.1. Deadline: Nov 1. Estimated annual cost: residents, $11,000; non-residents, $21,000. Public.

OHIO STATE UNIVERSITY

College of Medicine and Public Health

Admissions Committee

270-A Meiling Hall

370 West Ninth Avenue

Columbus, OH 43210-1238

In-state applicants: 1,345; out-of-state applicants: 2,601. Percent interviewed: 35%. First year enrollment: 134 men, 76 women. In-state acceptance rate: 80%. Average GPA: 3.6. Average MCAT score: 10.2. Deadline: Nov 1. Estimated annual cost: residents, $10,000; non-residents, $28,000. Public.

WRIGHT STATE UNIVERSITY

School of Medicine

Office of Student Affairs and Admissions

P.O. Box 1751

Dayton, OH 45401

In-state applicants: 1,250; out-of-state applicants: 2,137. Percent interviewed: 38%. First year enrollment: 40 men, 50 women. In-state acceptance rate: 83%. Average GPA: 3.5. Average MCAT score: 8. Deadline: Nov 15. Estimated annual cost: residents, $11,500; non-residents, $16,000. Public.

OKLAHOMA

UNIVERSITY OF OKLAHOMA COLLEGE OF MEDICINE

P.O. Box 26901

Oklahoma City, OK 73190

In-state applicants: 412; out-of-state applicants: 1,101. Percent interviewed: 45%. First year enrollment: 87 men, 61 women. In-state acceptance rate: 95%. Average GPA: 3.6. Average MCAT score: 9.2. Deadline: Oct 15. Estimated annual cost: residents, $8,000; non-residents, $19,000. Public.

OREGON

OREGON HEALTH SCIENCES UNIVERSITY

School of Medicine

Office of Education and Student Affairs, L102

3181 SW Jackson Park Road

Portland, OR 97201

In-state applicants: 371; out-of-state applicants: 1,752. Percent interviewed: 30%. First year enrollment: 56 men, 40 women. In-state acceptance rate: 71%. Average GPA: 3.6. Average MCAT score: 9.9. Deadline: Oct 15. Estimated annual cost: residents, $16,000; non-residents, $31,000. Public.

PENNSYLVANIA

ALLEGHENY UNIVERSITY OF THE HEALTH SCIENCES

MCP <> Hahnemann School of Medicine

(Formerly Hahnemann University School of Medicine)

Admissions Office

2900 Queen Lane Avenue

Philadelphia, PA 19129

In-state applicants: 1,303; out-of-state applicants: 9,554. Percent interviewed: 20%. First year enrollment: 119 men, 131 women. In-state acceptance rate: 50%. Average GPA: 3.3. Average MCAT score: 9.2. Deadline: Dec 1. Estimated annual cost: residents, $25,000; non-residents, $25,000. Private.

JEFFERSON MEDICAL COLLEGE

Associate Dean for Admissions

1025 Walnut Street

Philadelphia, PA 19107

In-state applicants: 1,247; out-of-state applicants: 8,732. Percent interviewed: 25%. First year enrollment: 135 men, 88 women. In-state acceptance rate: 39%. Average GPA: 3.5. Average MCAT score: 9.5. Deadline: Nov 15. Estimated annual cost: residents, $25,000; non-residents, $25,000. Private.

PENNSYLVANIA STATE UNIVERSITY

College of Medicine

Office of Student Affairs

P.O. Box 850

Hershey, PA 17033

In-state applicants: 2,000; out-of-state applicants: 4,894. Percent interviewed: 25%. First year enrollment: 59 men, 51 women. In-state acceptance rate: 54%. Average GPA: 3.5. Average MCAT score: 9.1. Deadline: Nov 15. Estimated annual cost: residents, $16,600; non-residents, $24,000. Private.

UNIVERSITY OF PENNSYLVANIA

School of Medicine

Director of Admissions

Edward J. Stemmler Hall, Suite 100

Philadelphia, PA 19104-6056

In-state applicants: 906; out-of-state applicants: 7,042. Percent interviewed: 17%. First year enrollment: 83 men, 67 women. In-state acceptance rate: 36%. Average GPA: 3.6. Average MCAT score: 11. Deadline: Nov 1. Estimated annual cost: residents, $27,000; non-residents, $27,000. Private.

UNIVERSITY OF PITTSBURGH

School of Medicine

Office of Admissions

518 Scaife Hall

Pittsburgh, PA 15261

In-state applicants: 1,024; out-of-state applicants: 4,254. Percent interviewed: 30%. First year enrollment: 65 men, 84 women. In-state acceptance rate: 58%. Average GPA: 3.5. Average MCAT score: 10.4. Deadline: Dec 1. Estimated annual cost: residents, $19,000; non-residents, $26,000. Private.

TEMPLE UNIVERSITY

School of Medicine

Admissions Office

Suite 305, Student Faculty Center

Broad and Ontario Streets

Philadelphia, PA 19140

In-state applicants: 1,217; out-of-state applicants: 7,061. Percent interviewed: 22%. First year enrollment: 114 men, 68 women. In-state acceptance rate: 66%. Average GPA: 3.3. Average MCAT score: 9.4. Deadline: Dec 1. Estimated annual cost: residents, $22,500; non-residents, $28,000. Private.

RHODE ISLAND

BROWN UNIVERSITY

School of Medicine

Office of Admissions

97 Waterman St., Box G-A212

Providence, RI 02912-9706

In-state applicants: 15; out-of-state applicants: 148. Percent interviewed: 4%. First year enrollment: 27 men, 39 women. In-state acceptance rate: 9%. Average GPA: 3.4. Average MCAT score: NA. Deadline: Mar 1. Estimated annual cost: residents, $26,000; non-residents, $26,000. Private.

SOUTH CAROLINA

MEDICAL UNIVERSITY OF SOUTH CAROLINA
College of Medicine
Office of Enrollment Services
171 Ashley Avenue
Charleston, SC 29425
In-state applicants: 558; out-of-state applicants: 1,955. Percent interviewed: 25%. First year enrollment: 80 men, 59 women. In-state acceptance rate: 94%. Average GPA: 3.4. Average MCAT score: 9. Deadline: Dec 1. Estimated annual cost: residents, $7,000; non-residents, $19,000. Public.

UNIVERSITY OF SOUTH CAROLINA
School of Medicine
Associate Dean for Student Programs
Columbia, SC 29208
In-state applicants: 433; out-of-state applicants: 911. Percent interviewed: 30%. First year enrollment: 44 men, 29 women. In-state acceptance rate: 97%. Average GPA: 3.4. Average MCAT score: 9. Deadline: Dec 1. Estimated annual cost: residents, $7,500; non-residents, $19,000. Public.

SOUTH DAKOTA

UNIVERSITY OF SOUTH DAKOTA
School of Medicine
Office of Student Affairs, Room 105
1400 W 22nd Street
Sioux Falls, SD 57105
In-state applicants: 138; out-of-state applicants: 859. Percent interviewed: 38%. First year enrollment: 25 men, 25 women. In-state acceptance rate: 99%. Average GPA: 3.6. Average MCAT score: 8.5. Deadline: Nov 15. Estimated annual cost: residents, $11,000; non-residents, $23,500. Public.

TENNESSEE

EAST TENNESSEE STATE UNIVERSITY
James H. Quillen College of Medicine
Assistant Dean for Admissions
P.O. Box 70580
Johnson City, TN 37614-0580

In-state applicants: 545; out-of-state applicants: 1,025. Percent interviewed: 32%. First year enrollment: 39 men, 21 women. In-state acceptance rate: 90%. Average GPA: 3.4. Average MCAT score: 8.7. Deadline: Dec 1. Estimated annual cost: residents, $9,000; non-residents, $17,000. Public.

MEHARRY MEDICAL COLLEGE
School of Medicine
Director of Admissions and Records
1005 D.B. Todd Boulevard
Nashville, TN 37208
In-state applicants: 245; out-of-state applicants: 4,663. Percent interviewed: 10%. First year enrollment: 41 men, 39 women. In-state acceptance rate: 15%. Average GPA: 3.1. Average MCAT score: 7.5. Deadline: Dec 15. Estimated annual cost: residents, $20,000; non-residents, $20,000. Private.

UNIVERSITY OF TENNESSEE
College of Medicine
790 Madison Avenue
Memphis, TN 38163-2166
In-state applicants: 610; out-of-state applicants: 1,147. Percent interviewed: 50%. First year enrollment: 100 men, 65 women. In-state acceptance rate: 87%. Average GPA: 3.5. Average MCAT score: 9. Deadline: Nov 15. Estimated annual cost: residents, $9,000; non-residents, $17,000. Public.

VANDERBILT UNIVERSITY
School of Medicine
Office of Admissions
209 Light Hall
Nashville, TN 37232-0685
In-state applicants: 321; out-of-state applicants: 5,517. Percent interviewed: 15%. First year enrollment: 67 men, 37 women. In-state acceptance rate: 18%. Average GPA: 3.7. Average MCAT score: 11. Deadline: Oct 15. Estimated annual cost: residents, $23,000; non-residents, $23,000. Private.

TEXAS

BAYLOR COLLEGE OF MEDICINE
Office of Admissions
One Baylor Plaza
Houston, TX 77030
In-state applicants: 1,196; out-of-state applicants: 1,772. Percent interviewed: 35%. First year enrollment: 96 men, 72 women. In-state acceptance rate: 73%. Average GPA: 3.7. Average MCAT score: 11.1. Deadline: Nov 1. Estimated annual cost: residents, $8,000; non-residents, $21,500. Private.

TEXAS A&M UNIVERSITY
College of Medicine
Associate Dean for Student Affairs and Admissions
College Station, TX 77843-1114

In-state applicants: 1,290; out-of-state applicants: 124. Percent interviewed: 30%. First year enrollment: 29 men, 35 women. In-state acceptance rate: 92%. Average GPA: 3.5. Average MCAT score: 9.3. Deadline: Nov 1. Estimated annual cost: residents, $8,000; non-residents, $21,000. Public.

TEXAS TECH UNIVERSITY
School of Medicine Health Sciences Center
Office of Admissions
Lubbock, TX 79430
In-state applicants: 1,479; out-of-state applicants: 81. Percent interviewed: 40%. First year enrollment: 78 men, 40 women. In-state acceptance rate: 90%. Average GPA: 3.4. Average MCAT score: 9.3. Deadline: Nov 1. Estimated annual cost: residents, $8,000; non-residents, $21,000. Public.

UNIVERSITY OF TEXAS - GALVESTON
Medical Branch at Galveston Office of Admissions
G.210, Ashbel Smith Bldg.
Galveston, TX 77555-1317
In-state applicants: 2,371; out-of-state applicants: 712. Percent interviewed: 40%. First year enrollment: 113 men, 87 women. In-state acceptance rate: 96%. Average GPA: 3.5. Average MCAT score: 9.3. Deadline: Oct 15. Estimated annual cost: residents, $7,000; non-residents, $20,000. Public.

UNIVERSITY OF TEXAS - HOUSTON
Medical School at Houston
Office of Admissions, Room G-204
P.O. Box 20708
Houston, TX 77225
In-state applicants: 2,401; out-of-state applicants: 852. Percent interviewed: 35%. First year enrollment: 122 men, 78 women. In-state acceptance rate: 96%. Average GPA: 3.4. Average MCAT score: 8.7. Deadline: Oct 15. Estimated annual cost: residents, $8,000; non-residents, $21,000. Public.

UNIVERSITY OF TEXAS - SAN ANTONIO
Medical School at San Antonio Admissions Office
Health Science Center
7703 Floyd Curl Drive
San Antonio, TX 78284-7701
In-state applicants: 2,385; out-of-state applicants: 770. Percent interviewed: 42%. First year enrollment: 105 men, 95 women. In-state acceptance rate: 92%. Average GPA: 3.6. Average MCAT score: 9.3. Deadline: Oct 15. Estimated annual cost: residents, $7,000; non-residents, $20,000. Public.

UNIVERSITY OF TEXAS - SOUTHWESTERN
Southwestern Medical School
Office of the Registrar
5323 Harry Hines Blvd.
Dallas, TX 75235-9096

In-state applicants: 2,325; out-of-state applicants: 861. Percent interviewed: 30%. First year enrollment: 149 men, 51 women. In-state acceptance rate: 87%. Average GPA: 3.6. Average MCAT score: 10.3. Deadline: Oct 15. Estimated annual cost: residents, $7,000; non-residents, $20,000. Public.

UTAH

UNIVERSITY OF UTAH
School of Medicine
Director, Medical School Admissions
50 North Medical Drive
Salt Lake City, UT 84132
In-state applicants: 414; out-of-state applicants: 843. Percent interviewed: 48%. First year enrollment: 69 men, 31 women. In-state acceptance rate: 75%. Average GPA: 3.5. Average MCAT score: 10.5. Deadline: Oct 15. Estimated annual cost: residents, $7,000; non-residents, $15,000. Public.

VERMONT

UNIVERSITY OF VERMONT
College of Medicine
Admissions Office
C-225 Given Bldg.
Burlington, VT 05405
In-state applicants: 106; out-of-state applicants: 6,963. Percent interviewed: 18%. First year enrollment: 43 men, 50 women. In-state acceptance rate: 40%. Average GPA: 3.4. Average MCAT score: 10. Deadline: Nov 15. Estimated annual cost: residents, $16,000; non-residents, $29,000. Public.

VIRGINIA

EASTERN VIRGINIA MEDICAL SCHOOL
Office of Admissions
721 Fairfax Avenue
Norfolk, VA 23507-2000
In-state applicants: 837; out-of-state applicants: 4,818. Percent interviewed: 25%. First year enrollment: 55 men, 42 women. In-state acceptance rate: 72%. Average GPA: 3.3. Average MCAT score: 9. Deadline: Nov 15. Estimated annual cost: residents, $16,000; non-residents, $26,000. Private.

VCU/MCV
School of Medicine
Medical School Admissions
MCV Station Box 980565
Richmond, VA 23298-0565
In-state applicants: 946; out-of-state applicants: 3,758. Percent interviewed: 27%. First year enrollment: 97 men, 73 women. In-state acceptance rate: 72%. Average GPA: 3.3. Average MCAT score: 9.5. Deadline: Nov 15. Estimated annual cost: residents, $11,000; non-residents, $25,000. Public.

UNIVERSITY OF VIRGINIA

School of Virginia

Medical School Admissions Office

Box 235

Charlottesville, VA 22908

In-state applicants: 837; out-of-state applicants: 3,637. Percent interviewed: 15%. First year enrollment: 86 men, 53 women. In-state acceptance rate: 72%. Average GPA: 3.6. Average MCAT score: 10.2. Deadline: Nov 1. Estimated annual cost: residents, $10,000; non-residents, $22,000. Public.

WASHINGTON

UNIVERSITY OF WASHINGTON

School of Washington Admissions Office

Health Sciences Center A-300, Box 356340

Seattle, WA 98195

In-state applicants: 995; out-of-state applicants: 2,193. Percent interviewed: 30%. First year enrollment: 91 men, 85 women. In-state acceptance rate: 88%. Average GPA: 3.6. Average MCAT score: 10. Deadline: Nov 1. Estimated annual cost: residents, $8,000; non-residents, $20,500. Public.

WEST VIRGINIA

MARSHALL UNIVERSITY

School of Medicine Admissions Office

1542 Spring Valley Drive

Huntington, WV 25704

In-state applicants: 274; out-of-state applicants: 773. Percent interviewed: 35%. First year enrollment: 30 men, 18 women. In-state acceptance rate: 98%. Average GPA: 3.5. Average MCAT score: 8.2. Deadline: Nov 15. Estimated annual cost: residents, $9,000; non-residents, $20,000. Public.

WEST VIRGINIA UNIVERSITY

School of Medicine Office of Admissions

Health Sciences Center

P.O. Box 9815

Morgantown, WV 26506

In-state applicants: 264; out-of-state applicants: 864. Percent interviewed: 80%. First year enrollment: 61 men, 25 women. In-state acceptance rate: 95%. Average GPA: 3.6. Average MCAT score: 8.6. Deadline: Nov 15. Estimated annual cost: residents, $8,500; non-residents, $21,000. Public.

WISCONSIN

MEDICAL COLLEGE OF WISCONSIN

Office of Admissions

8701 Watertown Plank Road

Milwaukee, WI 53226

In-state applicants: 420; out-of-state applicants: 6,101. Percent interviewed: 20%. First year enrollment: 126 men, 78 women. In-state acceptance rate: 55%. Average GPA: 3.5. Average MCAT score: 9. Deadline: Nov 1. Estimated annual cost: residents, $14,000; non-residents, $24,000. Private.

UNIVERSITY OF WISCONSIN MEDICAL SCHOOL
Admissions Committee
Medical Sciences Center, Room 1250
1300 University Avenue
Madison, WI 53706
In-state applicants: 545; out-of-state applicants: 2,014. Percent interviewed: 20%. First year enrollment: 78 men, 65 women. In-state acceptance rate: 86%. Average GPA: 3.6. Average MCAT score: 9.5. Deadline: Oct 15. Estimated annual cost: residents, $14,000; non-residents, $20,000. Private. Public.

Appendix B

Checklist for the Admissions Process

As you prepare for medical school admissions, be sure to keep up with any requirements or credentials you need in order to be as qualified as you can be. Don't wait till the last minute. Materials returned by AMCAS do not meet deadline requirements. The following is a checklist you should be familiar with from the start.

_____ Discuss career plans with your premedical advisor.

_____ Outline a 4-year curriculum that includes all the premedical requirements you'll need for entrance, a broad range of liberal arts electives, and some writing classes.

_____ Become involved in school and community activities as soon as possible, preferably during your freshman or sophomore year.

_____ Fall, junior year: Begin studying for the MCAT.

_____ Late-Winter, junior year: Register for the MCAT and return the application before the deadline.

_____ Early-Spring, junior year: Take the MCAT

_____ Early-Spring, junior year: Have all transcripts sent to AMCAS.

_____ Mid-Spring, junior year: Arrange to have letters of recommendation or a composite letter of recommendation sent to individual medical schools.

_____ Mid-Spring, junior year: Send in AMCAS application as soon after June 1 as possible but before school deadline.

_____ Summer, junior year: Send in all non-AMCAS materials, along with appropriate fees.

_____ Fall, senior year: Application deadlines for all individual medical schools.

Appendix C

Checklist for Registration and Application Dates

Activity	Deadline
Register for the MCAT	
Send in AMCAS Applications (names of schools)	
Send in non-AMCAS Applications (names of schools)	

Appendix D

Summary of Extracurricular Activities

Fill in the following activities as you do them because you may forget some. Refer to this list when filling out your application and writing your autobiographical sketch.

School Extracurricular Activities   **Dates**

_____

_____

_____

_____

Community and Social Activities   **Dates**

_____

_____

_____

_____

Volunteer Work   **Dates**

_____

_____

_____

_____

Employment (full and part time)   **Dates**

_____

_____

_____

_____

Academic Achievements and Awards   **Dates**

_____

_____

_____

_____